Surviving Cancer with Proton Therapy:
Road to Nami Island

York L. Phillips

with

Curtis Poling

First Edition - Copyright © 2012 York L. Phillips

ISBN-13: 978-0615645360

Published by York L. Phillips, St. Simons Island, Georgia, USA

Design and layout by York L. Phillips

Editing by Eileen Leunig and Sherrye Gibbs

Cover photograph by Tracy Poling

Printed in the United States of America

This book is designed to provide accurate information with regard to the subject matter covered. This information is given with the understanding that the authors are not engaged in rendering professional medical advice. Since the details of each patient's situation are different, individuals should always seek the services of competent professionals.

DEDICATION

This book is dedicated to the many men who have suffered, are suffering, or will in the future suffer from prostate cancer. This book is also dedicated to the many men, women, and children who will suffer from other localized cancers and who might benefit from proton beam therapy. I hope this book encourages cancer patients to take initiative on their own to understand their diseases, to fully understand the information they get from their doctors, and to explore the practical and available treatments.

Finally, this book is dedicated to the families and close friends of those with cancer. They suffer from cancer as well. I hope this book helps those who are close to cancer patients to understand the disease and the treatments and to be in a better position to give support.

May God be with you.

York L. Phillips with Curtis Poling

CONTENTS

FOREWORD - Dr. Cho

Prostate cancer in the early stage is highly curable. However, once you are diagnosed with prostate cancer, you will be scared and confused even if you are told you have an early stage of the disease. Then you will be overwhelmed by the flood of unrefined information from many different sources. You will be more frustrated and exhausted after hearing conflicting opinions even from different medical professionals. Eventually, you may have to start a long journey on your own.

This is the story of a gentleman who takes a long journey to research the best cure for cancer while maintaining his quality of life. Finally, having found proton beam therapy, he makes another long journey to Korea to receive treatment. I believe he made the right decision because proton therapy is potentially the best for similar situations.

The authors describe vividly what happens to the patient when he finds out that he has cancer and how it affects his loved ones. They also describe in a compassionate manner the vigorous process of searching for answers and the patients' journey, which ends in finding hope and happiness. Certainly, this book will well guide you on what to do if you or your loved ones have prostate cancer and want to avoid surgery.

Dr. Cho Kwan Ho (Dr. Cho)
Radiation Oncologist
National Cancer Center
Seoul, South Korea

FOREWORD - Mr. Jin

I would like to thank all of the people who had been successfully treated with the proton beam therapy in Korea. I would also like to extend my gratitude to Mr. York L. Phillips and Mr. Curtis Poling who have written this book, "Road to Nami Island", and Mr. Han Man Jin, President of KMI International, and his staff members who have orchestrated the proton beam cancer therapy project from the initial stages, as well as the medical tourism specialists in Korea for their full support. As you may know, Korea's top-quality level of medical science is comparable to or surpasses that of advanced countries. Korea has the highest percentage of cutting-edge medical equipment in the world, and yet, the cost of medical treatment is much lower than that of advanced countries. Korea certainly has a bright future in the field of medical tourism. Furthermore, as the representative organization responsible for promoting Korea's cultural content around the world, including top-quality medical services, the Korea Tourism Organization has been working in compliance with the government's policy on nurturing the medical tourism industry, which the government considers to be a new growth engine. Currently, the KTO has 28 branch offices abroad engaging in local marketing activities.

Danish futurist, Rolf Jensen, is known all over the world and has predicted that when the "Information Age" is over, the "Dream Society" will begin, which will provide stories, dreams, and emotive experiences to consumers. In the "Dream Society", medical tourism services in Korea will be based on a notion of warm-heartedness, sharing and communication, which will have a positive impact on many people all over the world. The emotive and touching stories in the book "Road to Nami Island" will surely give the patients dreams that all of the diseases which seemed incurable can be cured in Korea.

The KTO is putting forth its best efforts to become an efficient, challenge-driven, and harmonious organization in the 21st century. We are endeavoring diligently to make Korea a worldwide, warm-hearted and prominent medical tourism destination. I ask for your continuous interest and cooperation not only regarding proton beam therapy, but also in the field of medical tourism.

Thank You

Mr. Jin Soo Nam (Mr. Jin)
Executive Director
Korean Tourism Organization (KTO)
Seoul, South Korea

PREFACE

I started writing a novel a few years ago and told all my friends, including Curtis and Tracy, about my project (which is still on the back burner). Later, after Curtis returned from getting proton beam therapy at Loma Linda University Medical Center in California, he told me about his efforts to help men with prostate cancer discover proton beam therapy and the benefits of being treated at the National Cancer Center in Seoul, Korea.

I said "you need a book."

He said "why don't you write one?"

Over the last nine months, I talked to Curtis many times about his story. I also read his research and talked to several of the men he had helped get to Seoul. I also talked to his daughter, who is now helping him with his efforts to serve cancer patients.

I was in my local branch library during the period I was working on this book, and decided to see what the library had to offer in terms of books on prostate cancer. There were two books on the shelf. The card catalogue showed that the regional library (covering several counties) only had fourteen books on the subject. While these books appeared to be well written by doctors, some were less useful because they were old and the information in them was out of date. Even as I did research on the Internet, I found that not every website has the most up-to-date information. I started out to try to tell a story to help put a more human face on the process men go through in addressing this disease. In the course of working on the story, however, I concluded that part of my objective was to present a study guide to help people conduct research on their own and make informed decisions affecting their own condition.

Let's be clear: I'm not a doctor and I haven't personally experienced cancer. This book is intended to be a guide for learning about the topic and making informed decisions. There are many sources of information on the Internet, some of which are referenced here, as well as many other books on the subject. You will never be able to read and digest it all. Your information will come from websites, blogs, books, doctors, and others who have lived the experience. With this book I hope to help you learn how to gather and evaluate all the information in order to make the appropriate decision for your own situation.

Also the book may sound like I'm an advocate of a particular therapy. I am. I support the patient's careful consideration of proton beam therapy as it appears to be effective and to minimize the risk of very difficult side effects.

Proton beam therapy appears to be appropriate in many, but not all, cases. I also support careful consideration of having your therapy at the National Cancer Center (NCC) in Seoul, Korea, primarily because of the lower cost, the relative quick access you can have to obtain treatment, and the overall quality of care you will receive.

Having admitted these biases up front, I would direct you to Chapter 9 and the five points I am trying to stress: consideration of proton beam therapy is the fourth and consideration of the NCC in Korea is the fifth. More important than these are first: early detection by regular PSA testing for all men; second: learning to understand the meaning of the test results by working closely with your doctors; and third: maintaining a good general understanding of health issues.

Please note that, while the book is listed as non-fiction, the main storyline is fictional. From my research, the story tracks the process many people go through as they find out about cancer and (with the help of their families) develop and implement their own personal plans of action to deal with it. Fiction allows me to concisely present several scenarios, including prostate cancer among men and pediatric cancers. Hopefully this style will be suitable for adults and even for mature young people, who might need to know some more about the disease and the treatment that a family member is facing.

Finally, the topic of cancer and cancer treatment is evolving dramatically in this age of rapid technological change. In recognition of this, we have established a website to provide additional information and updates.

The address of this website is www.RoadToNamiIsland.blogspot.com. This reference is repeated at the end of most chapters in the section listing websites and other sources.

York L. Phillips
St. Simons Island, Georgia
May, 2012

ACKNOWLEDGMENTS

I wish to thank Curtis Poling, who gave me the idea for the book and told and retold his story many times as I wrote. Curtis also facilitated much of my research through discussions with other men who had received proton beam therapy. In this respect, I view Curtis as being significantly more than just a source.

I would also like to thank Noh Kyong-Tae (Mr. Noah) and Yang Eunjin, his wife, for their assistance in obtaining and verifying the descriptions of Korea.

I would like to thank the team of friends and relatives who helped me with my English, and particularly Sherrye Gibbs who did the final editing and my sister-in-law, Eileen Leunig, who thought she had retired from the book editing business. Based on the help they gave me, it was clear that I should have paid more attention in my high school English classes.

And finally, I would like to thank my wife, Vicki, for her patience and support as I worked on the book. I'll finish redecorating the bathroom as soon as I can.

COVER PHOTOGRAPH

The four gentlemen are all former prostate cancer patients who received proton beam therapy. The three on the left (from the left: Alfred Vismer, Douglas Atherley, and Hans van Roijen) received their treatment at the National Cancer Center in Seoul, Korea. The man on the right is Curtis Poling who was treated at the Loma Linda University Medical Center in Loma Linda, California. Following his treatment, Mr. Poling took the initiative to help other men with prostate cancer find out about the benefits of proton beam therapy. Subsequently, he became an advisor to the National Cancer Center in Korea to assist those with prostate cancer and other cancers obtain treatment at the National Cancer Center. The men in the cover photo are attending a reunion of cancer patients and are on a day-trip to Nami Island.

CHAPTER 1. JOE, THE AVERAGE GUY

Joe is not entirely an average American even though he started out that way. He was born and raised in Peoria, Illinois. His father worked for Caterpillar building engines for giant earthmovers. Joe was good in math and science in high school and was interested in mechanical things. He was especially fascinated by the machines his father built. He decided to go to college and pursue a career in mechanical engineering. He enjoyed engineering so much he decided to stay around to get a master's degree in civil engineering.   After college, he served in the US Army Corps of Engineers and then went to work for Caterpillar. That was pretty much where the "average" ended.

After five years, just before he turned thirty, Joe was struck by wanderlust. He felt the need to explore the world before he settled down. He had a plan. He fully expected that his urge to travel would end in a few years (he privately gave himself five) and that he would return to Peoria, find a nice girl, settle down, and finish his career by working at Caterpillar.

Joe traveled to South America and went to work for a contractor who was a major customer of Caterpillar. The contractor assigned Joe to the headquarters office in Argentina, but he also worked in Chile, Peru, and Brazil. Joe worked hard and enjoyed what he did. Time passed, and soon he realized that the five years in his original plan had stretched to nearly twenty. At the end of twenty years Joe was fifty. He left the contractor, took his pension in a lump sum and invested it, and hung out his shingle as an engineering consultant to the construction industry.

The contractor had developed a nice niche business working in several countries. It seemed that when one particular country was going through a political upheaval or economic downturn, some other country was resolving its political issues or experiencing economic growth. In addition, many projects were governmental in nature and those were often less affected by poor short-term economic conditions. As a result of his experience with the contractor, Joe had many contacts in the construction and development industry throughout major parts of South America. He used these to his advantage and did well in his consulting business.

By American standards, Joe did not make a lot of money, but the cost of many things in South America was much lower and Joe did well, relatively speaking. He also invested his pension wisely, and calculated that he would be able to live comfortably, even in the United States once he was ready to retire. Finally, he realized that he was young and healthy enough to practice as a consultant for a few years after he moved to the United States. At least, he thought, until his daughters were finished with college.

Oh yes, his daughters.

While he worked for the contractor, Joe had met and married a nice Argentinian lady named Maria and they had two daughters, Victoria and Teresa. Joe made no secret of the fact that he would eventually like to move back to the United States. Joe's wife and daughters loved it when he talked like this, as they very much approved of the idea of living in America. The general plan was to retire and move to Peoria in time for the girls to finish high school there, become acclimated fully to American culture, and attend college.

After five years in the consulting business, Joe was nearing fifty-five, and Maria was forty-five. Their daughters were in good schools in the equivalent of the eleventh and ninth grades. Joe was beginning to feel the urge to retire and return to the United States. He and the family had traveled many times to the United States over the years to visit family and to see the country. The girls had been to Disney World in Florida, New York City, and New Orleans, along with many other exciting places. Now they were beginning to think seriously about where they might go to college.

When he had left the contracting company, Joe had been dropped by the company's health plan. As an expatriate in Argentina, Joe's only option for health care was a private insurance plan. As Argentinian citizens, Maria and the girls were covered by the national health care program and by a trade-group program associated with Maria's job at the school library.

Joe had purchased a basic insurance plan. For one thing, he had found that the cost of healthcare was considerably less than he understood it was in the United States. For another, he and the family were all in very good physical condition. He kept a portion of his retirement nest egg in a separate account to be available in case it was needed, but so far he had not had to go into that fund.

One Friday afternoon as Joe was wrapping up his week's work, he received a phone call from the office of Dr. Silva, his family doctor. While he had decided to carry only basic insurance, Joe was especially careful with prevention. He and the family had thorough annual physicals to identify problems while they could be treated efficiently and successfully (and cheaply). It helped that in Argentina, medicine was more oriented to prevention than to the treatment of a disease after it was already established. Until he got the call, Joe almost forgot that he had recently gone to Dr. Silva for his annual physical.

"We have all your test results back and would like to schedule the follow-up for your physical as soon as possible. Can you come in Monday?" asked the receptionist.

Joe checked his calendar.

"Yes, how about 3 o'clock?" Joe asked as he scribbled the appointment in in his date book.

"That would be fine," replied the receptionist.

Joe cleaned up a few minor items on his desk and left for the weekend. His part time assistant had been out that day, so it was up to Joe to turn off the lights and lock the door. As he walked down the hall, it struck him as a little unusual that the doctor's receptionist had said that the doctor wanted the follow-up visit "as soon as possible." Normally, things were not urgent with the doctor.

By the time he got home, he had forgotten all about the call and was focused instead on plans for the evening.

Joe and his wife were scheduled to attend a reception at their tennis club as the kick- off for a teen charity tournament. The girls were scheduled to play in the tournament, and Maria was on the organizing committee. Joe expected to see his good friend, Bill, there along with Bill's wife, Rosario, as their son was also scheduled to play in the tournament.

When they got to the club for the reception and had finished the obligatory chore of going through the receiving line, Joe looked around for Bill and spotted him with Rosario. He took Maria by the hand and led her over to where they were waiting. As they arrived where Bill and Rosario were standing, a waiter came by and offered them glasses of Chardonnay. The four friends stood and chatted for a while.

They slowly separated into two conversations, even as they stood together. Maria and Rosario had gone to school together and had known each other long before they met their husbands. Their conversation touched on the tournament, the progress of their children in school, and on arrangements for their next family get-together - a picnic generally planned to take place a few weeks hence, but without a set date.

Bill and Joe had met and become fast friends soon after they had both arrived in Buenos Aires and before they met their wives. Bill worked for a branch of an American bank that had been established in Buenos Aires but after a few years had gone to work for an Argentinian bank that was interested in opening branches in some key cities in the United States. While their paths didn't cross from a professional point of view, their social lives had. They were lonely during that time and frequented clubs and often double-dated. They privately referred to themselves as the "Lonely Bulls" after the Herb Alpert song.

Bill had met Rosario at a reception honoring the bank's opening of a branch bank in another city. They had talked and discovered that they had common interests in art and music. Bill asked Rosario out and she had said she preferred it if they could include her friend Maria. Bill called Joe and recruited him to join them. They went to dinner and to a concert, and by the end of the evening both couples knew where their relationships were headed.

Bill and Rosario got married first, and Joe and Maria followed suit a few months later. At the reception following the second wedding, Bill and Joe made a ceremony out of retiring a small stuffed toy bull Bill had found.

During the evening, Bill mentioned that he had received a call from an old college roommate who was having a medical problem and needed Bill to come to Miami to help him deal with it.

"It's funny," Bill said. "I have had very little communication with Dennis over the years, even though we were the best of friends in college. I was his best man when he and his wife, Barbara, got married. About the most communication we have now are the Christmas cards we send to each other every year. For many years, we have recycled the same two cards - I send Dennis one and he sends me the other, then the next year we reverse them. But we did solemnly agree when we were in college to be available for each other in case we were ever needed. In any event, even though now is not the best time what with the tournament and winter vacation coming up, I made my airline reservations and will be leaving tomorrow night to fly to Miami."

Joe thought about this some and had a momentary uneasy feeling remembering how the doctor's receptionist had sounded more insistent than he would have expected.

The night's program proceeded to the part where the club's president thanked all the sponsors, the participants, the representatives of the charities that were to benefit, the committee that arranged the tournament, the moms and dads of all the players, and everyone else under the sun. Then it was finally over and Joe could go home.

As they waited at the club entrance for the valet to bring their cars, Joe asked Bill "Are we still on for lunch on Tuesday?"

"I don't know," Bill replied. "I am scheduled to go to Miami tomorrow night and to return overnight on Monday night. That gives me almost two full days there with Dennis and Barbara. I should be able to find out what's going on in that amount of time, but there's no guarantee. If I get back early Tuesday we can probably still meet for lunch, but I'll have to have Rosario call you and let you know."

Joe indicated that this would be fine.

Saturday and Sunday passed quickly. The girls were itching to practice for the tournament, but they each had a couple of important tests to take during the last week before the winter break was scheduled to begin. Maria and Joe had insisted that they put the tournament out of their minds for the time being and focus on studying. Joe pointed out that the tournament was not scheduled to begin for another two weeks and that there would be plenty of practice opportunity during the winter break.

On Saturday afternoon Joe volunteered to go with Rosario to take Bill to the airport for his trip to Miami. He wished Bill luck and again had a twinge of uncertainty about his meeting with the doctor scheduled for this coming Monday.

On Monday, family life and Joe's work schedule returned to near-normal following the relatively hectic pace of the weekend. The girls headed off to school fully prepared for their respective tests, looking forward to getting past the ordeal so they could concentrate on the vacation and the tournament. Maria said she would be busy the next couple of weeks, not only with the tournament committee, but at work. The library was scheduled to move into a new wing during the winter break and she was involved in the move. When construction started, the wing was supposed to be ready before the start of the school year in March, but Joe could look at the project and tell that this wouldn't happen. Once the new building was ready, the move was rescheduled during the vacation to avoid disruption to the students and teachers.

Joe went into his office and worked most of the day on the draft of a preliminary report based on his evaluation of a unique engineering design for a site to be occupied by a large industrial building. The issues related to a load-bearing analysis of the soils, as well as design of infrastructure (storm drainage, water and sewer lines, and access roads). He broke briefly for lunch and finished the report in the early afternoon. After his last proofing, he turned the draft report over to his assistant to proof once more, copy, and send out to the client.

His appointment at the doctor's office was set for three, and the office was only a short distance away. He got there a little early and sat in the waiting room glancing at the old magazines and medical pamphlets scattered throughout the room.

Eventually he was ushered into the doctor's office, where the doctor sat behind his oversized desk, studiously perusing some papers.

"You look out of place, Doctor Silva," said Joe to try and break the ice. "I usually only see you in one of the examining rooms. Without your lab coat you look like you could be the president of a corporation or a high government official."

The doctor smiled briefly, then gathered up the papers and put them in a manila folder. Then his face took on a more serious expression and he began.

"Joe, I wanted to be sure to see you as quickly as possible. We've been doctor and patient for many years and have become reasonably good friends. I want you to be successful as much as I want to be successful myself. Your test results are by and large very good. You have maintained a steady weight and low blood pressure and low cholesterol, and you don't show any signs of emerging complications due to age."

Joe started to relax a little since so far this was pretty good news. He hadn't had any significant problems in the past and was not entirely sure what problems he might face in the future, but he would be happy if that part of his life waited a bit.

"There is one test we took that causes me a little concern, however," the doctor continued. "We do a test as part of the blood work called a 'PSA' test. It stands for 'prostate-specific antigen' and measures androgens in the blood. In your case the level is elevated, rather significantly. I checked your previous physicals. We have been using this test on you each year since you were fifty and it has never been anywhere near this high. I would like to get another blood sample before you leave and I'm going to rush it through the lab to see if it confirms the earlier test. Some things can affect the validity of the PSA test, such as having sex or riding a bicycle shortly before the sample is taken."

Joe asked the obvious question: "What is the PSA test used to detect?"

"Oh. I guess I skipped that part. Sorry. The test detects antigens that are given off by the prostate gland. In a normal prostate the test has a very low number. In a prostate gland that is distressed, however, the number is higher. The PSA test is not the only test. You may recall that I also did a digital rectal exam, as I have for each annual physical since you turned forty. I did not detect anything unusual with that exam. That exam can indicate if there is a problem, but if no problem is indicated, it does not mean that there isn't something that doesn't show up. In that exam, I attempt to feel if there is any roughness on the part of the prostate that can be felt from the rectum. Roughness indicates a problem, but not all parts of the prostate can be felt that way.

"The kinds of things that can cause a higher PSA level include prostatitis, which is an infection usually caused by bacteria. It can also be caused by a condition known as benign prostatic hyperplasia, or BPH, which is an enlarged prostate. Also, the PSA level can be elevated following intercourse. Finally, it can be an indication of prostate cancer. Please understand that a large percentage of high PSA tests do not necessarily lead to a final determination that cancer is present.

"I want you to see a urologist. He will examine you and will arrange any other tests. The other tests he will want to conduct will probably include a biopsy, where he will take several small core sections of the prostate gland to look at under the microscope. A pathologist with specific training in conducting this work will be able to identify if there are problems indicated by the biopsy. If he finds any indication of cancer, he will also analyze it for what is called a 'Gleason score,' which gives an indication of the aggressiveness of the disease."

By now Joe was sweating and getting fidgety. He had many questions, but couldn't really organize them into coherent, articulate thoughts.

"I know you are concerned," Doctor Silva continued more soothingly. "As I said, there are several conditions that could be responsible for a jump in the PSA level. We will take another blood sample now and have it analyzed to see if this might have been just an anomaly. But we want to be careful, because one of the possibilities is prostate cancer. And that doesn't necessarily mean there is an immediate problem. About two-thirds of prostate cancer cases involve very slow growing cancers. A large majority of men in their eighties, for example, have prostate cancer but will die of another cause before the cancer affects them. You are young, however, in terms of this disease, and we need to evaluate the situation and make the right choices for you. You are also in very good physical condition. We may have identified this problem early, which is always a plus in solving it. In fact, we don't really yet know if there is a problem. I want you to see the urologist and have these additional tests. I have already arranged for them. I hope you are free Wednesday afternoon to meet with the urologist."

"Yes. Of course," was all Joe could muster. Then he asked "what was the PSA amount and what should it be?"

"The PSA was 6. There is no real normal, since it varies from man to man, but it is generally considered that the range of 0 to 4 is normal. In addition to a high number, however, we look for dramatic changes. If a man generally has a PSA around 1 and it jumps to 3, that might indicate a problem. Your PSA a year ago was around 1. But we still have much information to gather. Now come with me to the lab so the technician can take some blood."

The doctor's technician drew a blood sample, and Joe left, still a little stunned.

Normally, Joe took the bus to work and home again, not so much because the bus was convenient and cheap (although it wasn't bad), but because the rush hour traffic was such a pain. On this day, however, Joe was not up to finding the bus and fighting the crowds. He was still blown away by what he had learned. Instead, he hailed a cab (which was in itself a matter of luck) and gave the driver his home address.

"Perhaps," he thought to himself "finding a free cab this quickly in rush hour is a sign." He sighed and reminded himself that reading signs wasn't the best way of handling the situation.

The cab found some lucky breaks in the traffic and got Joe home in a near-record twenty minutes.

Joe's mind was still spinning, and he hadn't even thought of how he was going to approach the task of breaking the news to Maria.

Before he turned the door knob he took a deep breath and straightened up. He always found that part of approaching a difficult situation was having a positive attitude, and part of having a positive attitude was in the posture he assumed.

The girls were in their room finishing their homework. Maria was in the kitchen putting the finishing touches on something that was headed into the oven. He smelled a roast and knew that what was still to be cooked was a side dish. She heard him come in the door and came out to give him a peck on the cheek.

"Don't let me touch you," she said. "I'm just about finished preparing dinner and my hands are dirty. Go change and pour us each a glass of wine."

Joe suddenly realized that he had more questions. For example: are you supposed to refrain from drinking or are you supposed to drink more? He remembered reading about a study that said a glass of red wine was the best thing to have. Just like the studies that alternately said coffee would kill you or it would make you healthy.

After he changed, Joe came out and selected a bottle of Argentine Malbec wine that he and Maria had found in one of their trips into the country. Joe was pleased with the improvement in the quality of Argentinian wines over the last several years, which had led to increased exports. He poured two glasses just as he heard the oven door close and the little chirps that indicated Maria was setting the timer.

They sat down in the living room while the TV news droned on in the background.

Before Joe could speak, his wife said "I got a call from Rosario. Bill called her from Miami and plans to take a flight that leaves this evening and arrives early tomorrow morning. He told Rosario that he is still expecting to meet you for lunch tomorrow. He said since he'll be up all night, he might sleep in when he gets here, but if the lunch can be a little late, he'll make it. She also said that Bill junior is having a case of nerves for the tournament this weekend. I don't see any sign that Victoria is going to be affected by nerves."

Just then, the girls burst out of their room yelling "homework finished! Hi, Daddy, what did you bring us?"

This was an old joke. When they were little and Joe had to travel a lot on business, he always found some trinket or gift to bring. Soon it seemed that they were only interested in the gifts and not in his return. Maria was the first to figure it out, and thereafter his instruction was not to bring anything home but that as soon as they could after his return, they would go out for a special family dinner at one of their favorite restaurants. The girls figured it out, however, and the family joke was the "what did you bring us?" line.

Joe relaxed a little. He turned off the TV that no one was watching and flipped on the radio to his favorite easy-listening radio station. The girls automatically turned up their noses and acted like this was "old people" music.

"Time for dinner," said Maria, coming in from the kitchen.

They washed up and went into the dining room. While they ate breakfast and lunch at every time under the sun and in every odd location, the rule was that the family would eat dinner together as often as could be arranged. When they instituted the rule, referred to as "Rule 1," the girls moped and acted insolent because they were missing their favorite program on TV or just "had" to call a particular friend, so they instituted "Rule 2," which was that each person had to tell something new and interesting that happened to him or her that day. This included the parents, and everyone got to vote to make sure that a story was not boring or repeated from a recent night. Again, this became something of an unnecessary tradition as the girls always had many new things to tell and were itching to get their turn to "present."

Once the prayer was given and the roast served (this was Argentina, after all - beef country!), the competition for story-telling began.

Victoria started with what her tennis coach at school had told her. He had given her hints about how to approach the upcoming competition. She wanted to go over to the courts and try a few things out. Everyone agreed that this would happen on Wednesday, since the girls got out of school early and Joe could take them.

Teresa was next, telling about what she learned in geography class. The class was studying Asia and the "Pacific Rim," and this month's focus was on Korea. She told what she had learned about the results of World War II and the Korean Conflict, and the Demilitarized Zone and the talks at Panmunjom.

Maria recounted her conversation with Rosario about Bill's return after visiting his old college roommate. She didn't include the part about Billy being nervous about the tennis tournament, not so much because Victoria might play against him (they were in different age groups), but she didn't want to give Victoria the notion that there was something to be nervous about.

It came to Joe, and he realized that the big news he had wasn't something he was ready to tell. He needed to talk to Maria first. So he quickly went to his backup idea and told about finishing the report on the construction design for the industrial project.

Three dinner napkins flew his way. This was the signal, based on football officials in American football throwing the flag for a "personal foul," and indicated that this report was a loser. The girls and Maria got a kick out of how much Joe liked American football, since they had no use for it or any clue as to why anyone would watch it. "It's too complicated," they said. "See how simple and elegant real football is?"

Joe would simply respond "We're going to move to the United States and you're going to attend college. If you don't understand American football and know when to cheer at a game, how will you ever get a date? Hmmmm? Anyway, if you think this is complicated, how will you ever understand baseball?"

The arguments long ago became a tradition and a jovial family sport.

After dinner, the girls checked their homework with Joe and Maria while the dishwasher did the dishes. After that the girls were free to call friends and watch TV until bedtime, and Joe and his wife retired to the living room.

Joe sighed. Now was the time to tell Maria what happened, and he steeled himself, not so much because he thought he'd get a bad reaction but because he simply didn't like to deliver bad news.

"I went to see Doctor Silva today," he began. "You know I just had my physical two weeks ago and the doctor wanted to go over all the results with me."

Maria smiled and put her hand on his knee. So far this sounded pretty straight forward.

"How was everything?" she asked.

"Generally good. In fact except for one issue - one possible issue - I did really well." So far this wasn't as hard as he had prepared himself for.

"My PSA level is high, and the doctor is concerned about it." He proceeded to relate the full conversation in the doctor's office, while Maria listened intently.

"So," she said slowly when he was finished "they want to do some more tests because they are not sure there is actually anything wrong?"

Maria had a way of getting down to the core of the situation and putting a positive spin on it. Maybe Joe was being more alarmed than he needed to be at this point. He always appreciated his wife's maturity and calm demeanor.

"Yes. I think you could look at it that way. You know, all my life I've never really had any kind of serious medical problem. I have had colds and the flu, and all the normal childhood diseases except the mumps, but nothing that was really more than an inconvenience."

Maria thought a moment, and then spoke carefully. "It sounds to me like we need to take this one step at a time and develop and follow a plan. You're a good engineer with lots of experience. Let's approach this the way you would a big engineering project, like the one you tried to put over on us a dinner." She giggled, and Joe had to smile.

"Well of course, you know that the only reason I did that was that I wasn't ready to come out with the big news." But he was smiling too.

"OK. I understand perfectly. Let's be logical; how would you approach this if this was one of your consulting projects?"

"Well," Joe answered. "Let's just go into our office and work it out that way."

The family had a spacious apartment in a convenient location near the girls' school and in a nice section of town. Maria worked during the school year at the school library, so it was desirable for her as well. They had chosen to live in an apartment and sacrifice yard space for the good location, making up for it with membership in the tennis and swim club and extensive use of the neighborhood parks. The location fit their lifestyle very well and they were very happy with it. "Let someone else mow the grass and weed the flowers," Maria would say.

The apartment had three bedrooms. Joe and Maria shared the master, and the girls shared the larger of the remaining rooms (actually, almost like a second master bedroom, with its own bathroom and large closets.) This allowed Joe to keep an office in the smallest bedroom. They had figured out early that this would help Joe stay at home and get work done when he was very busy, rather than having to go to his downtown office on nights and weekends. The family appreciated this trade-off, preferring to have Joe at home in exchange for giving up a little space. And the girls didn't seem to mind sharing a room.

In exchange for the consideration, Joe willingly agreed to share the office with Maria for use as her office. The room was also equipped with a small convertible sofa for use as a guest room by their infrequent guests.

The office had desks and permanent computers for each of them, along with a TV and radio. On one wall, Joe had installed a whiteboard that he used when he needed to think and outline a particular problem and conceptualize a solution.

Joe cleared a space on his work table. He had used it to gather information for his latest project during the last couple of weeks but he was finished with most of the materials now. He had not spent any time in the home office over the weekend as he was busy with the tennis tournament, but he had finished the draft of the report today and could put away his research. He also erased the whiteboard, ready for the new project.

"Okay. Where shall we begin?" He stared at the board. "To start, I don't know the first thing about cancer in general or the prostate gland or prostate cancer. I don't know what the prostate does. I don't know what causes prostate cancer. I don't know what it does to you. I don't know how it can be treated or what the prognosis is." He noted the list of questions on the whiteboard.

"You left out something," said Maria, thoughtfully. "You don't know if you even have it."

"Good point," he said and drew a line and added that point. "Which, of course, also suggests that we don't really know how it is diagnosed."

Soon they had put together their basic plan for research and turned to their computers to proceed.

The first place they went was Google to look up prostate and prostate cancer and were referred to several websites. They looked at several articles on Wikipedia. They each read the articles two or three times, since it had a considerable amount of information and used many unfamiliar words. Eventually they got the basic idea, and Joe put a second list on the whiteboard:

- cancer - usually slow developing (2/3 of cases)
- men later in life - most men older than 75/80 have it, but many die of other causes
- detection - PSA screening and others (digital rectal exam)
- treatment strategies - surgery, radiation, "wait-and-see," chemotherapy, hormones

They followed most of the links from the articles and added a few more lines of notes. About midnight, Joe yawned and announced that he couldn't think straight any longer.

"So far," Maria commented, "I don't think we have found anything that is particularly disturbing. I still contend that you need to find out more about what is happening in your case."

Joe agreed.

They went to bed and hugged. Soon he heard her gentle snoring.

Joe reviewed his day. Often when he was facing a difficult situation he would go through a routine before he went to sleep. The routine was based on his training as an engineer, but he could apply it to personal problems as much as he would apply it to technical, engineering problems. Essentially the routine consisted of considering what the situation was and what he knew; what the alternatives might be for an outcome; what other things were going on that might affect the outcome or might affect his ability to deal with the situation (he referred to these as the external factors); and finally, he would fix his mind on an outcome that was positive. This last step didn't necessarily solve the problem, but it helped him put his mind at ease so that he could fall asleep without worry. He referred to this last step as his sleep spin.

In this case, he determined that he did not know very much about the situation with his PSA results and would need to learn a lot more over the next few days. As to alternatives, he knew from his brief research this evening that it could mean anything from an anomaly in the testing up to and including prostate cancer. As to other factors, he was a little bit concerned over the situation Bill was going through with his friend Dennis. Again, he did not have much information but was gratified that he might be able to find out tomorrow if Bill could keep their lunch date. At least this issue might be out of the way.

Another external factor was Maria. He realized he was much more upbeat about this situation now that he had started doing something about it and knew he had his wife's support. He realized that her stability and common sense would get him through this trial as much as anything else would. He thanked his lucky stars (as he had many times in the past) that he had Maria for a wife. Whatever happened, Joe considered himself halfway to victory over any problem because of her love and support. He focused on this thought for his sleep spin.

Websites Joe and Maria used to get general information on the prostate

Note: for updated information on websites and other information in this book, please see www.RoadToNamiIsland.blogspot.com.

http://men.webmd.com/picture-of-the-prostate

http://en.wikipedia.org/wiki/Prostate

CHAPTER 2. PROBLEM IN THE PROSTATE

The next day, Tuesday, Joe delayed his departure for the office. He had finished his preliminary report on the construction investigation and had left it for his part-time assistant to copy, collate, and mail. He made a call to Rosario to see if Bill had returned as planned.

"Yes. He rolled in about eight this morning. He's sleeping now, but he said he got some sleep on the plane and would be able to meet you about 2 PM. He suggested the restaurant next door to the tennis club."

This was good, since it was closer than trying to go to the office and then turning around to go to lunch. He called his assistant and said he probably wouldn't be in at all but would work from home. He got a list of the phone messages and returned the calls. He also called two or three people about the construction review project and told them that the draft preliminary report was on its way to them.

At 1:15 he left for the club. For mid-winter it was a pleasant, almost spring-like day, so he decided to walk. As he walked, he realized he was a lucky man. He had a wife and family he loved and good friends like Bill and Rosario.

He arrived before Bill did and secured a table in a quiet corner with a view of the outside patio. The patio was normally lined with greenery, but in the winter was without significant flowering vegetation and was not used by the diners.

Bill arrived only a few minutes after Joe did. He looked worn out as he approached the table, and the normal bounce was missing from his step. But of course he had just spent all night on an airplane and two days with a friend who was apparently in some kind of trouble. Joe and Maria had discussed how Joe should handle his friend, and Joe decided to let Bill dictate the pace of the discussion. He had told Maria, however, that he was going to fill Bill in on his own situation if it appeared to be appropriate. Bill was too good a friend to withhold information from.

Bill started. "Well, you look almost as tired as I feel. What have you been up to?"

"Put it on me right away," Joe thought to himself. This is not the way he had planned it.

"I was up late last night doing some research. Never mind about me, though. We can get to that later. Tell me all about your college roommate and what transpired this weekend."

Bill went through the whole story, starting from when he received the call on Friday.

His former roommate and best friend from college, Dennis, had just come from an appointment with a doctor and had received some bad news concerning his prostate cancer. He had tried to discuss it with his wife, Barbara. She wasn't able to handle it very well, but he needed to talk to someone. Dennis was in a position professionally where he would have to keep any bad news like this quiet or risk losing clients, and many of his close friends were also clients. He needed to talk to someone who could be discreet. When he noticed Bill's Christmas card on the bookcase next to the desk in his home office, he immediately recalled their pact in college to always be available for each other. That's when he decided to call Bill.

Joe had perked up when he heard prostate cancer. He had lots of questions.

"As soon as we finished our conversation I called the airline," continued Bill. "There were no seats on the Friday night flight, which is just as well, since I probably would not have made it to the airport in time. I was, however, able to book a seat on the overnight flight leaving here Saturday night. Of course you know this because you took me to the airport."

The waiter came and Bill paused in his story so they could order.

Bill resumed his account. "In any event I took the overnight flight, but at least it was non-stop and I got a little bit of sleep. I got into Miami Sunday morning and Dennis picked me up at the airport. We went to his house, which seemed to have a pall hanging over it. Dennis' wife, Barbara, had obviously been crying a good bit. Fortunately, they don't have any kids or anyone else in the house, so the mood hadn't spread. It was almost a surprise that the entire neighborhood wasn't gloomy, but Dennis really stressed that he needs this to be a secret for the time being. He has a couple of clients who actually live close by.

"Anyway, once we got to his house and settled in, Dennis gave me the whole story. Barbara apparently didn't even want to hear it. She left the room, went somewhere else in the house, and shut the doors.

"To start with, Dennis is about our age. We went through college and graduate school together and shared an apartment for a time before Dennis married Barbara. Dennis gets a routine annual physical most years. When he had his physical three years ago, his PSA was higher than normal; I think he said it was 13. The doctor took another sample and confirmed the result. Now I'm not really sure what a PSA test measures, but I learned from Dennis' story that it has to do with prostate cancer. Anyway, at that time the doctor told Dennis that while it was elevated, the PSA level wasn't particularly high, and the digital rectal exam he did at the time didn't indicate anything unusual. Also, the doctor mentioned that not all men had the same PSA level and that this might be normal for Dennis. The doctor then said that any problem would be slow to develop, and that the best approach for the time being would be to simply keep a close eye on the situation."

Joe thought that if this had been a week ago he wouldn't have known what a PSA test was either, but he kept quiet for the moment and listened to Bill.

Bill continued. "Dennis basically let it go. He missed his physical the next year because he had a business deal he had to work on, but since the previous year the doctor had said just to watch it, he didn't think this would be a problem. That would have been two years ago. The next physical he had was last year. His PSA level was at 18, which was higher than it had been the first time. The doctor gave him a digital rectal exam and said it didn't indicate anything abnormal. Again, he told Dennis that any problem of this type was typically slow in developing and that the best strategy was to keep any eye on it, but he suggested that Dennis see a urologist anyway. He gave Dennis a referral and Dennis said he would do that."

Their lunches came and they went about eating. Joe had not eaten a very big breakfast and realized he was hungry. He hoped he wasn't feeding a cancer; he had heard the expression, but realized he didn't really know what it meant.

As they ate, Bill continued the story. "Dennis put off making an appointment with the urologist until a few months later when he saw a news report on TV about September being 'Prostate Cancer Awareness Month.' This was September last year. He made the appointment and finally went to see the urologist in November last year. When he made the appointment, the doctor's office had him get another blood test, which he did. The urologist told him that his PSA level was still higher than it had been in previous tests. I think he said it was at 28. He examined Dennis and gave him another digital rectal exam, and told him that the PSA test was the only indication that there was a problem. He explained to Dennis that he was concerned about a pattern of increasing PSA levels, indicating that the tests were probably not anomalies. He said he didn't agree with Dennis' regular doctor that it should simply be watched, but that he would not know exactly what the problem was unless there were further tests. He recommended a biopsy and explained that this would involve an outpatient procedure to take samples from his prostate that would be examined by a pathologist to determine if there was any sign of cancer.

"Dennis was not particularly worried by this, since both his doctor and the urologist had described any problem as being typically slow to develop and his doctor had said the best strategy was to keep an eye on it. He arranged with the urologist for a date for the biopsy, but delayed it a couple of times due to conflicts in his schedule. He finally had the procedure earlier this year, in January, I think. I don't know too much about biopsies, but I think he told me that they took twelve cores or samples, and that two of them showed cancer.

"Anyway, a few days after the biopsy he met again with the urologist. He said that the pathologist's analysis of the biopsy had concluded that the staging was relatively low and that he had a Gleason score of 3 plus 3, or 6, and that it indicated that the cancer was not too severe. I'm not sure exactly what staging means, but it appears that these numbers all have to do with the seriousness of the disease. The doctor told him that, based on the report from the pathologist and his own evaluation of the biopsy slides, he believed the cancer is a 'garden variety' case. He said that Dennis was a good candidate for several different treatments.

"He told Dennis that there were a couple of forms of radiation therapy, including x-rays and some kind of treatment where they implant radioactive seeds in the prostate to kill the cancer cells. He said that Dennis would be a good candidate for these treatments, and that he would also be a good candidate for surgery, where they remove the prostate itself. Finally, he told Dennis that other therapies, including chemotherapy and hormone therapy, were not indicated because of the relatively early stage of his disease and the lack of any indication that it had spread. He told Dennis that he recommended surgery, that surgery was a well-established form of treatment, and that he could perform the surgery with a minimum of delay. He said that there are side effects and consequences of all of the forms of treatment that were available. He said that the side effects of radiation included the possibility of secondary cancers being caused by the radiation. He described the side effects of surgery as including the possibility of some loss of bladder control and/or sexual function, but that in Dennis' case the surgery looked fairly straight forward and he didn't believe that there would be any significant complications. He also didn't give any statistics to indicate to what extent the side effects appeared as the result of different forms of treatment.

"Dennis spent a few days, thought it over, and discussed it with Barbara. His impression at this point was that surgery would be the best course of action. Based on the doctor's recommendation and descriptions of the side effects of the various treatments, he was not particularly interested in chemotherapy or radiation. Dennis said he knew or had heard of people who had had these treatments and had been ill as a result. He elected to have the surgery. He had the surgery about a month later, as he had to give his own blood a few times to build up a reserve for use in the surgery.

"The doctor also arranged for Dennis to have an MRI to confirm if there were any possible complications before the surgery. He told Dennis that the MRI did not indicate any spread of the disease."

The waiter cleared their plates and took their order for coffee. The lunch crowd had largely cleared out and they had the restaurant pretty much to themselves.

"Dennis had the surgery in late February," Bill continued, "after donating some of his own blood to be used in the operation. Barbara had waited at the hospital during the surgery and had seen Dennis soon thereafter in the recovery room. She told me later that she was horrified at Dennis' condition when she saw him. She said 'He was weak and limp and pale, with tubes running into and out of him all over. From what he told me the doctor said, I never expected that.'

"The urologist (who was the surgeon) met with Dennis in the recovery room and told him that there had been a few complications. He said he had to remove some lymph nodes and some nerves because there was an indication that there had been some limited spread of the cancer, but he believed that all of the cancerous tissue had been removed. He explained to Dennis that he would need to be catheterized for a month.

"Dennis stayed at home for a month to recuperate, although he was itching to get back to work and still expecting everything to return to normal. Dennis had a blood test a few days before his second follow-up visit which was scheduled in June, just over three months after the surgery. When he met the doctor, he was told that his PSA was higher than was expected, and that it should have been close to zero. The urologist explained that the PSA level indicated that the surgery might have missed some microscopic cancer cells, called stem cells, and that there was a chance that these cells had spread. He arranged for Dennis have a bone scan to determine if there was any indication of the disease spreading.

"Dennis had the bone scan a week later, and it showed some lesions on the bones. Dennis returned to the doctor's office to consult over the findings of the bone scan. The doctor discussed possible additional treatment with radiation or chemotherapy. He expressed concern however, that radiation might not get all the cancer cells if they had already spread. Dennis was still not inclined to have radiation or chemotherapy, for the same reasons he gave before. That is, he knew people who had suffered ill effects from these treatments.

"As an alternative, the doctor suggested hormone therapy to reduce the level of PSA, but explained that it would not actually kill the cancer cells. Instead, it would delay any advance of the cancer. He also said it would prolong Dennis' life.

"When he left the doctor's office, Dennis was very upset. His understanding all along had been that this was a relatively benign and slow-evolving disease and that the disease and the surgical treatment were very routine, with a high rate of success, and a good long-term prognosis. In Dennis' mind, radiation and chemotherapy were treatments used for serious cancer cases, and that he was not going to need these. Finally, he was surprised at the mention of death. Death had been suggested only as the remotest of possibilities, and now it seemed almost inevitable.

"And so this was the point when he called me."

Bill explained that while he was there, Dennis and Barbara were alternately depressed and angry. Bill couldn't really do anything for them because he did not understand the disease or the natural human reaction (including the basic stages of grief), so he listened to them a lot.

"What I can't really get over was their anger," concluded Bill. "On the return flight, I jotted down some notes so I would remember what I heard."

He pulled a folded envelope out of his pocket. "In a nutshell, Dennis and Barbara were angry at the doctor and the urologist for soft-pedaling the disease and the need for treatment. They weren't completely sure, but based on the little they had read and learned, any cancer (like any other disease) can best be treated if it is caught early. They felt that the delays and the suggestions that it was okay to wait were not the correct advice. They were also angry at the urologist for apparently down-playing the effects of the treatment. Dennis had to be catheterized and could no longer achieve an erection. Barbara was very upset about this, because they had had a good sexual relationship up until the surgery. Finally, they were now concerned that Dennis might actually die, while very little had been said to them before indicating that this was more than a very remote possibility."

They sat quietly for a few moments, each thinking his own thoughts.

"Well," said Joe, finally. "That's a lot to ponder."

Joe was so engrossed in Dennis' situation that he had forgotten his own.

Bill brought him back to earth very quickly.

"So, what have you been up to?" asked Bill.

Now Joe needed to disclose his own news to his friend. He realized that Bill was worn down by the experience with Dennis and Barbara, but Bill would be upset if Joe didn't tell him. Making the story as upbeat as he could, he explained his own situation and what had transpired over the last couple of days.

When he was finished, Bill exhaled. "Phew. One would almost think that I might be a jinx with two of the people I care about the most coming down with the same malady and me finding out about both of them at the same time. Is there an epidemic going around that I haven't heard about?"

Joe closed the conversation. "Well, remember, I have not been diagnosed yet, so don't get too far ahead in worrying about me until I have more concrete information. Anyway, I have always believed that things will work out, and I have that confidence right now. I'll fill you in after I get more information. Tonight it sounds like I'm going to be doing some web surfing again this evening."

Bill chuckled. "That's one of the differences between you and Dennis. When the subject is something outside of his area of expertise, he kind of sits around and waits for things to happen to him while you go out and tackle the situation, no matter what it is."

They talked a little bit about the tennis tournament, which would occupy their families for the next week and a half. When they paid the check and left to go their separate ways, they agreed to keep each other informed.

Joe made dinner for the girls and put aside some for Maria. She was becoming concerned that the committee that was running the tournament was not on schedule to get things done and felt she needed to take a more active role so that there would be no complications. Accordingly, she made sure she would attend all the remaining meetings so that she would be able to do what she could to help keep things going.

After dinner, Joe returned to his computer and researched prostate cancer treatments and their side effects, following up on what Bill had relayed from Dennis' story. He was careful to keep a list of all the sites he went to so that Maria could repeat the process when she had her chance.

One other thing Joe did was to look for books on the subject, so he went to Amazon and searched under prostate cancer.

Joe found that there was a large number of books, some of which were available as downloads through Kindle. He had no idea which books would be helpful to him and which ones would not. He used a technique that he found useful in other situations. He read as many of the reader reviews as he could with particular focus on the reviews that were labeled as the "best of the bad reviews." While he was not ready to select and purchase any books, he started to get an idea of the range of issues reflected in the reviews. Among other things, he discovered that there were different camps representing opinions on the types of treatment available. Some books and some readers favored surgery, while others favored different forms of treatment. He made a list of books that looked promising for further research.

Maria got home about ten that evening. They sat in the kitchen while she ate, and Joe repeated Bill's saga. He included what he told Bill about his own situation and described what he had said to try to keep Bill upbeat.

"Sounds like Dennis' wife, Barbara, needs some hand-holding help." Maria suggested.

"Not all women - or men for that matter - are as mature and helpful as you are," said Joe. He sighed. "I just hope and pray that things do work out. I have faith they will. I know you just ate, but let's go to bed. It's been a long day and I'm really tired. I have the meeting with the urologist tomorrow." He explained the surfing he had done and the list of books he had identified. He told her that he had emailed her a list of the sites he had studied along with the book list.

"I have to be at the school library in the morning, but I'll check all that out as soon as I get home."

In bed, she murmured "If you do have prostate cancer, I hope there is a treatment that doesn't involve inability to have an erection. Of course I want you alive and healthy first."

"And we don't want incontinence either," he added.

She made a face.

Maria was soon snoring lightly, but Joe lay awake for a while, thinking about a number of things. He thought about Dennis and Bill's description of Dennis' anger at the doctors and the way they had soft peddled the information they gave him. He thought about his own situation and the duty he had to maintain a stable environment for his wife and the girls. He knew that if anything happened to him, they would be okay, but he wanted to be there to continue helping the girls grow up and he wanted to grow old with Maria. After a while, he searched around for positive thoughts, and decided to focus on a positive outcome of whatever treatment he might find appropriate to use, if it became necessary to do so. Surely, while he was finding cases of prostate cancer that were uncomfortably close to home, there must be cases with positive outcomes. Eventually, he went to sleep.

The urologist was located in a medical complex not far from Doctor Silva's office and his appointment was not scheduled until 2 PM, so Joe took the regular bus to his office and did some clean-up work. He took a taxi to the urologist's office, arriving in plenty of time. The doctor was running behind schedule, so Joe had to wait. None of the magazines appeared to be newer than three or four months, and he was not in the mood to read medical flyers and magazines anyway, so he settled on an old tennis magazine and thumbed through an article on South America's best tennis resorts.

"Maybe someday I'll take Maria and the girls to one of those," he thought, and added wryly, "if I get the chance."

Eventually he was ushered into an examining room and the doctor breezed in.

"Good afternoon, sir," he started, glancing at the thin file.

"I see this is our first consultation. I have examined your records, including the PSA test results and the result of the blood sample you gave on Monday. The PSA does not appear to be an anomaly. In fact, it has risen a little since the earlier test, which was" he paused, shuffling papers "almost three weeks ago."

He proceeded to give Joe a digital rectal exam, listened to his heart and lungs, and poked around in general.

"Have you noticed any change in urination, with respect to frequency, urgency, or flow? And do you find that you need to get up more frequently at night to urinate?" he asked.

Joe thought a minute.

"Well, yes," he said slowly. In fact, he had noticed that he needed to go to the bathroom more often and had to get up several times a night to go. He had also noticed that the urge to urinate came over him rather suddenly at times. But when he went to the bathroom he sometimes couldn't go very much.

He told all this to the doctor, who peered at him over his glasses.

"Have you noticed any blood in your urine or found it to be painful to urinate?" asked the doctor. "And have you experienced pain when ejaculating?"

Joe said he had not and experienced a brief glimmer of hope.

"Have you had any difficulty achieving an erection, that is, more difficulty than normal?" the doctor asked.

Again, Joe thought the question over, but wasn't sure how to answer.

"On a scale of one to ten, how easy has it been to have an erection?" the doctor clarified.

"On a scale of one to ten," responded Joe, "if it used to be eight or nine, they are now four or five. That's real subjective, of course."

"No, that's very helpful," said the doctor. "Most men don't keep score, and there are no real standards to measure by."

Joe smiled, "I guess not."

"When you insert, can you hold the erection?"

"Sometimes I won't stay erect as long as I used to." These questions caused Joe to think back. How long had some of these conditions been going on? He decided that this was only over the last few months. He told himself that this was probably a good sign.

"Okay. I don't see any indication that we need a CT scan or an MRI yet, but we are going to schedule a biopsy. Are you familiar with these procedures?"

Joe said he had a general idea what the CT scan and MRI were, but was not familiar with the specifics of what the biopsy would involve. His doctor had given him a very brief explanation, but by no means detailed.

"OK," said the urologist. "For the biopsy, we will use local anesthesia and insert a device in the rectum that will take a small core sample from the prostate. We will need to do this several times in order to get samples from several different parts of the gland. This way, if there is a problem we are more likely to find it. I couldn't find anything with the digital exam I just performed, but that's not unusual. When we do the biopsy, we will use a sonogram to make sure we hit the right areas.

"Once we collect the samples, we will have the pathologist look at each one under the microscope. If he finds evidence of cancer cells, he will let us know. He will also tell us which samples were positive. Knowing where the different samples were taken, we will have a better idea of the location of the cancer cells. Finally, the pathologist will rank the cancer on what is called the Gleason score. To do this, he will assign a score of 1 to 5 to the sample which appears to be the most involved, and likewise he will assign a 1 to 5 score to the second most involved sample. He will add these two scores together to get a total score, which will be between 2 and 10.

"Also, if cancer is found, we will develop a score, known as staging. This is a shorthand way of describing the extent of the cancer. This score can be used in communicating information and watching any changes. The score is made up of three components and is called the TNM system, with each letter representing a component. In short, the 'T' component describes the local extent of the tumor itself; the 'N' component describes the degree of spread to nearby lymph nodes; and the 'M' component describes the degree of spread otherwise, known as 'metastasis.' If you're interested, I can give you some websites to research for more detail.

"To prepare for the biopsy, you will need to do several things. The most important is that you will not be able to use aspirin or other blood thinners between now and the biopsy. Do you take aspirin now?"

"I take baby aspirin about four times a week," answered Joe.

"Ok. Stop taking them. I'll also give you a sheet of instructions on how to prepare for the biopsy. In order to let the aspirin clear out of your system, we will need to wait about three weeks before we conduct the biopsy. Did you bring your calendar?"

Joe nodded. They picked a date and the doctor called the receptionist to have her schedule the appointment.

"She will call you to confirm the appointment for the biopsy," added the doctor. "Make sure she has the correct phone number and knows the best time to call. Now do you have any questions?"

"I'm sure that as soon as I get out to the street I'll have a hundred questions, but right now I can't think of any," Joe told him.

Joe dealt with the receptionist and headed for home. Like Monday, the traffic was heavy and he took a taxi.

On the way home, he marveled that he was much calmer than he had been only two days earlier. He suddenly wondered how Dennis was.

When he got home, the girls pestered him and Maria to take them over to the tennis club to practice a little.

"We may as well," said Maria. "They've finished their tests and the next two days will be fairly unimportant as far as schoolwork goes."

To the girls she said "I suggest we go right now and put supper off a little bit. You don't want to play on full stomachs, and the demand for the courts will increase later so we're more likely to find a free court now."

At the tennis club, Joe and Maria sat in the bleachers and watched the girls play each other. There were only a few people at the club, this being the middle of the week and fairly early. The afternoon players had gone and the evening players had not yet arrived.

Joe had been noticing that Teresa was becoming a very good player, and nearly was the equal of Victoria.

"Teresa is going to be the one to get the tennis scholarship," he mentioned to Maria, who smiled and nodded.

Joe gave a complete account of the visit to the urologist, and Maria listened carefully.

"So the next step is the biopsy and for that we wait for - what was it - three weeks?" she asked.

"Correct," said Joe. "They need time to let the aspirin get out of my system. They gave me a sheet of other instructions. I won't be able to eat after noon the day before the procedure, and I have to take that drink that clears your system out. You know the one they make you drink before you get a colonoscopy. And on the day of the procedure I'll need to give myself an enema. And finally, I'll need to be brought home."

"Boy, you're a pretty demanding guy," said Maria with feigned reproach. "By the way," she added, "I looked at the list of books you compiled. I think it would help if you purchased one or two right now so you can learn a little more than we have been able to learn from the Internet. Maybe you can get Kindle editions so you won't have to wait."

Joe agreed that this would be a good idea.

The crowd was starting to come in, and the court had been reserved, so they gathered up the girls and headed home.

After supper Joe told Maria that there were a couple of things about the visit to the urologist that he wasn't clear on, so he went online and looked up prostate again and biopsy. Then he searched for information on Gleason score and staging. He also went back to Amazon and bought two books that he thought would include a good general overview. He bought hard copies rather than Kindle downloads but arranged for express shipment.

When Maria joined him, he showed her the results of his Internet searches and the books he had selected.

Maria nodded. "I guess the next big thing will be to get the biopsy taken care of and see what happens after that. I know you're going to be anxious until you get more information, but just be calm and relax and let's concentrate on having a good time with the girls for the next couple of weeks."

"I agree," he said. "No point in getting upset until there's more concrete information."

The next three weeks moved by fairly quickly. Joe was not pushing hard at work for new projects. He still had to work on the final report on the industrial development project, but he was waiting for the client's team to return comments on the preliminary report.

Some years the family took a vacation out of town during the winter school break. This was typically when they made their trips to the United States, because it was the middle of the summer there and a good time to travel. This year they hadn't planned anything special, particularly to leave time for the tournament preparation and the tournament itself. The tournament preliminary rounds were scheduled for the weekend that was in the middle of the break and the final rounds were scheduled for the weekend at the end of the break. A few of the parents had objected to this schedule, as they hoped to be gone for the entire two weeks, but most of the parents preferred to get the event over before resuming the busy school-year schedule.

On short notice, Joe took the family for a long weekend vacation to a rural vacation village during the first weekend of the break. They were lucky to get lodging for a few days at this late date, but they came across a small inn that had received a cancellation.

Joe's books from Amazon arrived the day they before they left on their short vacation, and he took them along to read. He shared much of what he learned with Maria.

They returned home on the Tuesday of the first full week of the winter break. The girls were anxious to get back to tennis practice, and Maria was still caught up in the moving of the school library. The movers had moved the boxes by the time she returned, and now everyone was busy sorting the books and putting them on the shelves. This task would take until the winter break was over.

As they got into bed the night they returned, Joe told Maria about some of the changes he was noticing in himself.

"Three weeks ago, I had no idea what PSA was, and the extent of what I knew about the prostate was that it had something to do with men's health, but I didn't know what. I was focused on working hard and achieving, and I'll have to be honest and admit that, while I love the family, there were times I was thinking more about work and achievement. On this little vacation I found myself looking at you and the girls differently, thinking about the things we have done and the things that make us happy. The other afternoon, when we were in the gift shop and you three were looking at jewelry, I actually looked at the pieces and the three of you and could see what made you happy. It's like this situation, whether or not it turns out to be cancer, makes you think about how you fit in with other people and makes you care more about the ones you love."

Maria didn't say a word, but hugged him until they both went to sleep.

On the Saturday of the preliminary tournament rounds, everyone was up early and ate a light breakfast. The girls had gathered all their equipment and were excited to get going. Even though the calendar showed that it was mid-winter, it turned out to be a fine spring-like day, with sunshine and only a few scattered clouds. The temperature was mild.

"The committee sure asked for and got Chamber of Commerce weather," Joe said, then had to explain to the girls what that expression meant. "It means it's the kind of beautiful weather that the Chamber of Commerce would like to have so that visitors to the community want to come live and open businesses."

"The committee was very careful about this point," said Maria, feigning seriousness. In fact, she was very happy about the weather.

The girls and Billy had matches scheduled at different times. Maria and Rosario would be tied up most of the time at the registration table checking in players, posting brackets and results. Joe and Bill had no official duties other than to cheer and to run errands for their wives. This they did very well.

Most of the time this left Joe and Bill with the opportunity to sit in the bleachers and talk. When they had one such occasion, Joe asked if Bill had heard anything from or about Dennis.

"Well, I won't hear anything about Dennis from anyone other than Dennis himself. That's just the way he is. I've called a couple of times and left messages, but I haven't heard back. I dare not call him at this office since he's so nervous about any of his clients finding out what's going on. As I understand it, he should have started the hormone therapy by now, but I really don't know. I may have to go up there in a couple of weeks to see if I can find out more. I am starting to worry. Dennis' parents died when we were in college and his brother died a few years ago. Barbara is the only family he has, as far as I know, and she's not able to give me much information.

"Speaking of Dennis, how's your situation? I haven't talked to you since, let's see, Tuesday. Didn't you go to the urologist?"

Joe told Bill all about the visit to the urologist, not leaving out any details.

After the Saturday afternoon and Sunday preliminary matches, the remaining players were seeded for the finals to be held the following Saturday. Both girls and Billy made it to the finals. All the parents were proud.

By Sunday evening, everyone was tired. Supper was pizza, a rare treat.

The first opportunity Joe and Maria had to talk again was Sunday evening when they went to bed.

Joe told Maria about his conversations with Bill, including what little he had learned about Dennis' status.

"I have some sad news," said Maria with sadness in her voice. "I haven't had you alone to be able to tell you. One of the parents told us this afternoon that Mr. Ruiz - you know him, he's on the board of directors for the club and used to be the treasurer - just passed away from prostate cancer. Apparently he didn't tell many people he had it and chose to have radiation treatment. The cancer not only spread, but he got additional cancer from the radiation treatment itself. Have you run across this situation in your research?"

"Not in detail," Joe replied, "But I think I have seen some reference to this. I'll follow up on it."

Maria, who was as tired as the girls, soon fell asleep.

While he was tired, Joe couldn't shake the image of Mr. Ruiz. Dennis' situation was bad, but Joe only knew Dennis by reputation. He had never met Dennis personally. On the other hand, he had been to many meetings and functions at the tennis club and had known Mr. Ruiz for several years. He had a hard time coming to grips with the idea that the man was no longer alive.

Because of these thoughts, he couldn't find a positive spin to place on his day. Eventually, fatigue took its toll and he fell asleep.

On Monday, Joe went to his office and took care of his mail and some phone calls. He was anticipating that he would get out early and go home to do some more research. Just before he was planning to leave, however, he got a call about his analysis of the industrial project. The client was happy with the report, but needed it to be completed as soon as possible so it could be submitted with a proposal for permanent financing for the project.

This would be no problem but would occupy Joe for a few days as he chased down all the remaining comments and assembled the final report. The client also wanted Joe to attend a meeting with the financial backers slated for the following Monday. Fortunately, the meeting would be held in Buenos Aires and would only last one day. He would not have to be away overnight and could be available for his biopsy appointment on Wednesday.

Joe made several calls to shake the trees and get the final reviewers to respond as soon as possible. He wasn't successful with everyone, but he did get the important ones to commit. He then compiled the comments he already had and made the necessary changes to the report. This activity took until Wednesday to complete, but by then he had received the remaining comments and was able to reflect on them. By the close of business on Wednesday, he had completed the final report, proofed it, had it proofed again by his assistant, had it copied and sent out to the local recipients by courier and to the out-of-town recipients by mail. He also scanned the report and emailed it to all the recipients so they could begin reviewing it before the hard copies arrived.

The next few days passed quickly. The girls went every chance they could to the tennis club or the park, depending on the weather. Maria told them to be careful not to get too tired in case it would affect their play on the weekend, but they seemed to have limitless energy.

Joe worked on the report, making changes as the comments finally started coming in.

Maria was busy with the library move and usually arrived home a little late. Joe cooked more meals than normal, but the girls loved his cooking because it wasn't so healthy.

In the evenings, Joe continued his Internet research. As he learned more about the subject of prostate he was able to expand his searches and learn even more.

"Hello," he said to himself one evening as he reviewed the information he had gathered. At this point, Joe realized that his research did not cover treatment options that well. He had been focused on what the problem was, or might be, but not on what can be done about it. Consequently, he adjusted his approach and started compiling a list of treatments. He realized that this was largely moot if it turned out that he had some other malady rather than cancer, but he preferred to be prepared.

On Friday, Joe's client on the industrial development called. He wanted a meeting with his team to prepare for Monday's meeting. Joe spent the day at that task.

By the weekend, Joe was tired of thinking. He was ready to watch some tennis and cheer.

The format was similar to that of the previous weekend. The girls and Billy had matches at various times. Maria and Rosario again had responsibilities at the official's table, but these were less demanding than they had been in the first rounds, so they were able to take turns and watch some of the matches themselves. Joe and Bill mostly sat in the stands and talked.

"Have you heard anything from Dennis?" asked Joe.

"I have," replied Bill. "He has started the hormone therapy and says he feels better. He is more upbeat about his prospects, but Barbara told me when Dennis wasn't on the line that the doctor says the situation is fairly serious. She asked me to be ready to come in case I was needed, and I told her I would."

They also discussed the situation with Mr. Ruiz. Bill knew him better because, as club treasurer, Mr. Ruiz had handled the club's bank accounts. Bill said he had been shocked to learn of his death.

"I was, too," said Joe. "Until now I realize that I have been able to view this whole situation in the abstract. Even the Dennis situation is entirely personal for me since I never met him. I feel close to it because you are so close to it, but still there is a layer of separation. On the other hand, I knew Mr. Ruiz as a real person, and it's hard to think of him as being gone." He waved his hand in a dismissive gesture when he said it, and Bill understood him perfectly.

"Maria found out more details this week," Joe continued. "He had surgery in April, and was told that the surgery was successful, but just a few weeks ago, he felt ill and was taken to the hospital. They discovered that the surgery had not removed all the cancer and it had metastasized and spread quickly throughout his body, and it killed him."

"Wow. That was quick," Bill exclaimed.

Joe was thinking through the timeline. Can you die of this cancer before you even know you have it? He thought of Dennis, and noted that Mr. Ruiz had surgery at the same time as Dennis. These were questions he needed to research and ask the urologist.

The tournament ended with final round losses by the girls and a win by Billy. Joe explained that this would help them to build character, but they were only partly happy. They asked him if this was the way they talked about American football, and Joe told them it was. They giggled.

Later, Joe confided to Maria that the girls had both done very well, considering that this was the first really big tournament they had been in.

By Sunday evening, everyone was tired and happy that it was over. Joe continued to be preoccupied thinking about Mr. Ruiz. After supper, Joe went into his home office and reviewed his materials for the meeting on Monday. Monday was also the first day of school after the winter break, so the girls and Maria got to bed early.

The meeting with the investors on Monday went well. The developer orchestrated the presentations on marketing, finances, design and construction, and feasibility. Joe was essentially there to say that the site development and building designs were sound and feasible and that there would not be any likely factors that would either delay the project or increase the construction cost or the cost of operating the finished product. Joes report was thorough and had been widely circulated. There were few significant questions.

While many of the participants retired to the bar at a nearby club to celebrate, Joe slipped out as soon as it was polite to do so and went home. He told the very happy developer client that he had been involved in the tennis tournament all weekend and was tired.

After supper, Maria and the girls, groaning about being back on the regular school-day schedule, were ready for bed early. Joe spent a little time in his home office researching prostate cancer therapies, but soon gave up and turned in early as well.

On Tuesday, Joe began his final round of preparations for the biopsy. He had restricted himself to a very light diet since Monday and to a liquid-only diet on Tuesday, including fruit juice and consommé. On Tuesday afternoon he began the regimen of drinking the liquid that would clear out his system. That afternoon and evening he remained at home near the bathroom.

On Wednesday, three weeks after meeting with the urologist, Joe presented himself at the urologist's office for his biopsy. Maria took the day off from work so she could accompany him and drive him home. The procedure was carried out by a specialist. Joe was a little suspicious because the fellow looked fairly young.

The specialist nodded and chuckled. "I've done dozens of these and haven't lost a patient yet. I'm going to hook up the sonogram so that we can make sure we are hitting the spots we need to take samples from."

He gave Joe a mild anti-anxiety drug and a local anesthesia and allowed them to take effect. When they did, he proceeded to take about a dozen samples, one at a time, placing each in a separate, pre-marked container indicting the location of the sample. As the process went on, Joe became more uncomfortable, but it was soon over.

Maria took Joe home. He went to bed. The urologist had told him that one of the side effects of the procedure was that he would be sore for several days; another was that he would have some bloody discharge in his stool, his urine, and in his semen for a couple of weeks. But this was the only definitive way to know exactly what the problem was and what the location and extent of the cancer was.

Websites Joe used to get more information about prostate cancer

Note: for updated information on websites and other information in this book, please see www.RoadToNamiIsland.blogspot.com.

http://en.wikipedia.org/wiki/Prostate_cancer

http://www.ncbi.nlm.nih.gov/pubmedhealth/PMH0001418/

http://www.pcf.org/site/c.leJRIROrEpH/b.5699537/k.BEF4/Home.htm

http://www.cancer.org/Cancer/ProstateCancer/OverviewGuide/prostate-cancer-overview-what-is-prostate-cancer

CHAPTER 3. THE BIG "C"

On Friday, two days after the biopsy, Joe and Maria had breakfast with the girls before they left for school. Normally, Joe would have left earlier to go to the office but today he was going directly to the urologist's office to get the biopsy test results.

The girls had noticed the odd schedule that had been in effect all week, what with Daddy not going in to the office as much and in the evenings he and Momma were in the home office concentrating on their computers. They were also dimly aware of Bill's travel to Miami a few weeks before. They were also aware that Bill and Daddy had been talking seriously a lot lately.

Notwithstanding, the tennis tournament was now over and they were focused on getting back up to speed with school and looking forward to the end of the school year.

"Why didn't you go to the office today, Daddy?" asked Victoria as she was finishing breakfast.

"Your Mom and I have an appointment and we decided to do that first," answered Joe. "Now don't be late for school."

After the girls left for school, Joe and his wife resumed their discussion over whether or not Maria should accompany Joe.

"I really think that this is a private matter and that the doctor might be a little hesitant to tell you everything you need to hear if I'm there," said Maria. "I'll be here and you can come directly back and tell me what happened."

"You're my partner and this affects you just as much as it affects me, maybe more. I've got an idea. Why don't you come and we can ask the doctor if he minds your sitting in? If he has a problem, you can sit in the waiting room and read old magazines."

The both chuckled. "Okay," said Maria. "That sounds like a good compromise. But remember, as soon as I see that he doesn't want to say something, I'm going out of the room."

"Agreed," replied Joe. "Anyway you can add a second set of ears and help me make sure I didn't miss anything. Also, if you can come in you can take notes on what is being said and let me concentrate on the discussion."

They kissed to seal the deal.

It was after rush hour and the traffic had died down to the normal midmorning mess. They drove to the oncologist's office with little trouble. They asked the nurse if she thought the doctor would mind if Maria accompanied Joe in to the appointment. The receptionist said she didn't see any reason it would be a problem, and that many people do that, but that they would need to ask the doctor.

Shortly, after silently leafing through the magazine selection, Joe was called into the doctor's office. He asked if Maria could come in, too, and the doctor said it would be okay.

"I have gone through all the tests, and I have talked with Doctor Silva, your family physician. Before I get into all the information, I'll answer your first question first: yes, your tests are positive, you do have prostate cancer. Now I'll get down to the details."

Joe exhaled and shifted a little in his chair. He glanced at Maria. Her expression didn't appear to change. He hoped he was right in encouraging her to come with him.

The doctor continued. "As I said, I have talked with your family physician and part of the reason I thought it would be not just okay, but good for Maria to come in with you was what he told me about the two of you. He said he hadn't seen many couples who were as mature partners as you two are. This disease affects the entire family, and the entire family needs to be involved in the process of overcoming the disease."

Joe had several thoughts in quick succession. First, he considered how Bill's friend, Dennis, and his wife had not appeared to do well at handling bad news. Second, he realized that asking Maria to come was a good idea after all. He stole a glance in her direction and saw that her expression had softened.

"Joe," the doctor said, turning from the two of them to speak directly to Joe. "Typically this particular kind of cancer is slow-growing and I am confident that it has not metastasized. We have identified it early which gives us more choices on what can be done. You are relatively young, as men with prostate cancer go. You are also in very good condition, as indicated by your recent physical exam. Consequently we will not choose a wait and see approach. If you were much older or otherwise in poor health, we might do that because of the typical slow growth of this type of cancer.

"I would like to select a program of treatment as soon as possible," continued the doctor. "We appear to have identified this cancer early and have a very good chance to be successful in stopping its growth. The chance of success diminishes, however, as time passes. Accordingly I would recommend that we get on with it.

"As I said before, I have discussed your case with Dr. Silva and I feel as though I know you, Joe. You have probably already done some research on treatment options, but let me review them for you. The first option is to do nothing, but we don't really have that option. As I indicated you are going to live longer than it will take for the cancer to become a problem, so we need to deal with it proactively. Therefore, we need to review the other options.

"One possible treatment is surgery, in which we go in and remove the cancerous tissue from the prostate. This may take the form of a prostatectomy, where we remove the entire prostate, or we may remove only a portion of the prostate or more than just the prostate if indicated by the spread of the disease. Surgery is the form of treatment that has been used longer than any other form of therapy for prostate cancer. We consider it to be the gold standard for treatment.

"Another treatment is external beam radiation, where we use doses of radiation focused on the cancer cells, essentially to damage them so they won't divide. This is done with x-rays. There are a couple of different types of x-ray radiation, the most innovative being IMRT, which stands for Intensity Modulated Radiation Therapy and involves the ability to deliver a more precisely aimed dose of radiation. This and other newer forms are essentially designed to be more accurate in targeting the tumor, thus allowing the dosage to be higher while doing less damage to adjoining healthy tissue.

"Another type of radiation therapy is known as brachytherapy, where we implant small seeds with radioactive material in the cancer. The radioactivity kills the cancerous cells and the level of radioactivity declines as the radioactive component of the seeds decays. The plan is to destroy the cancer cells within the effective life span of the radiation.

"There are other forms of treatment, such as chemotherapy, hormone therapy, and drug therapy, as well as some experimental treatments. These are generally not indicated unless the cancer has progressed. I would like to see if we can gain success quickly.

"We can also combine two or more of these forms of treatment into a program of treatment, selecting the correct combination based on a number of factors. These factors include the nature of the cancer, your age, and your overall health. Again, we appear to have identified the problem early enough that it hasn't had a chance to spread.

"In your case, Joe, I recommend surgery. As long as the cancer is confined to one location it will be easier to ensure that it has been completely eliminated. Also, you are in good overall condition and I believe you can withstand the surgery.

The doctor continued, getting a little more serious in his tone, "Now, you must understand that there are complications that can develop and that there are side effects of any form of treatment. For surgery, the location of the tumor makes surgery very difficult and requires great precision. Nevertheless, the surgery can damage other, nearby organs. More common side effects may include incontinence, as the bladder and urethra can be damaged, or erectile dysfunction."

These were the things Joe had read about and wanted to avoid.

"What about radiation?" asked Joe.

"Radiation does not involve physical invasion of the body," began the doctor, slowly. "We use x-rays that are highly focused to bombard the tumor in such a way as to damage the tumor cells."

"No, no, I understood what you said before," interrupted Joe. "What I meant was what about side effects of radiation treatment?"

"Of course," replied the doctor. "The x-rays damage any cells they pass through, including otherwise healthy cells on the way into the body and cells on the way out. They can also damage cells in the immediate vicinity of the tumor because the x-ray beam is not as precise as we would like. Damage to these healthy cells causes them to change and can actually create secondary cancers that weren't there to begin with."

Maria spoke for the first time. "Tell me more about what causes the erectile dysfunction."

The doctor smiled slightly and said "To put it in simple terms, there are bundles of nerves lying very close to the prostate. These nerves affect erection and can be damaged by certain kinds of surgery or radiation. In years past, these nerves were routinely removed during surgery to make sure the cancer had been completely removed. More recently, however, more refined surgical techniques and better control of radiation have reduced the chances that these nerves will be damaged. Be aware, however, that there is no guarantee that these nerves will not be damaged."

Joe thought about some of the numbers Bill had mentioned in connection with Dennis' situation.

"What are my PSA numbers and the numbers you obtained from the biopsy?"

"Good question," answered the urologist. "Your PSA has been hovering around 6 based on the last few blood tests." He referred to the file and continued "over the last few years your PSA was in the range of 1 to 1.5. The biopsy showed a Gleason score of 3 plus 3, or 6. This score is made up of an analysis of the first and second most involved samples, each of which is given a score of 1 to 5. Adding the 3 plus the 3 gives the overall score of 6. Finally, your staging is T1c, which is intermediate. This stage means the only indication we have so far is your PSA level. There is no indication of cancer from the digital rectal exams, nor do we have any evidence of any spread of the disease."

"These scores are the reason I say your cancer is fairly limited at this point and gives you more choices for treatment."

Joe had come across some of these terms in his research. He didn't know what Dennis' staging was or what his Gleason score was. He did recall, however, that Bill said Dennis' PSA was 13 and then had climbed to 18. He resolved to learn more about how these numbers are calculated and what they mean in practical terms.

They got a few more questions answered and Joe and his wife agreed to discuss the information and make a decision on the course of treatment no later than early the following week.

Joe had a sudden thought as they were going out of the office and turned to ask "In my research I came across someone using the expression 'don't go with photon, look into proton.' What might that mean?"

"There is a relatively new radiation treatment based on using a beam of proton particles as opposed to x-rays, which are photon beams. You can check out this therapy, but I don't have any information on it and have never treated a patient who used it. Anyway, it's generally not available outside of the United States. Also it's expensive and there are long waiting lists."

"Thanks. We'll check it out just the same," said Joe.

They shook hands with the doctor and left.

Now that he knew some more, Joe felt a little more stable, even though what he had learned was not good all news.

"Do you want to stop and get lunch?" he asked Maria.

"No. I heard a lot that I didn't know yet and I'm itching to get home and get on the computer and learn some more. I don't think we know enough yet."

Joe was glad that he had an ally in Maria. He loved her very much.

They got home and made sandwiches and a pot of coffee, then booted up their computers.

They made some quick notes on the whiteboard about the paths they would pursue in their Internet research. They did not want to repeat any searches unnecessarily, but they wanted to make sure they didn't leave out anything important.

"You take Google, and I'll take Yahoo," said Joe. "We'll search the same terms and compare what we get. That'll give us an idea of the places to follow up with more thoroughly. We can go through each page of each linked website and note the ones that appear worth following up on, and then we can go back through the ones we identify and get the information. We can each open a word processor file and copy the useful-looking links over to it."

"Sounds like a plan," said Maria.

"Let's start back at the beginning with the search terms we have already used," suggested Joe. "That way we will note everything and make sure we didn't miss something along the way."

They went to work. The idea behind Joe's strategy was to get a broad sense of the universe of sites that might have useful information, narrowing it down to those with the best and most complete information. This would avoid the temptation to jump around from website to website, finding information but not being able to analyze it thoroughly. By midafternoon they had amassed a fair list of websites to pursue. They discovered that by each taking a different search engine they had many duplicates but there were instances when one found some information that the other did not get.

After searching for prostate they searched for prostate cancer and prostate cancer treatment. After they reviewed the basic information on prostate, prostate health, and prostate cancer, they concluded that they had not learned much that they had not already covered in previous web searches or from the various doctors. They changed their focus to start addressing specific treatments. They referred to the list Maria had made on her notepad when they were in the doctor's office and compared it to several of the lists that they had gathered from websites.

They cleaned off the whiteboard and made a master list by compiling the several lists they had developed from the online data:

traditional types:
- "watchful waiting"
- surgery (radical, etc.)
- external radiation (x-ray)
- Cyberknife (another form of external radiation)
- internal radiation (brachytherapy)
- hormone therapy
- chemotherapy

new types:
- cryosurgery - "freezes" cancer
- biologic therapy
- high intensity focused ultrasound (HIFU) - "cooks" cancer
- proton beam therapy

The major differences among the articles seemed to be how detailed they were in the various types of the different treatments. Also, some treated proton beam therapy as experimental, while others did not.

Joe moved it up on the list, which then looked like this:

traditional types:
- "watchful waiting"
- surgery (radical, etc.)

- external radiation (x-ray)
- Cyberknife (another form of external radiation)
- internal radiation (brachytherapy)
- proton beam therapy
- hormone therapy
- chemotherapy

new types:

- cryosurgery - "freezes" cancer
- biologic therapy
- high intensity focused ultrasound (HIFU) - "cooks" cancer

After Joe and Maria put the basic list together they reviewed it. They had identified several articles to read in Wikipedia, as well as a number of websites and blogs to explore. At this point they each pursued part of the list, letting the other know when an article looked particularly interesting or useful. They each opened another document in the word processor and kept notes on the useful information and the source.

The process allowed them to cover a considerable amount of material efficiently in a short period of time. The afternoon wore on and they finished the first round of research on the individual therapies. When the girls got home they realized that they had lost all track of time, so they took a break.

Having made no arrangements for supper, they decided to order pizza. This was more than fine with the girls.

After they ate, they sat around the table giving their daily reports. Joe pretended to be interested but his mind was elsewhere.

"How did your appointment go? You know, the one you stayed home for," asked Victoria.

Joe and Maria glanced at each other and Maria answered quickly "We took care of it. We have something to tell you, but we don't have all the information yet, so it's too early."

"Are we going to have another sister?" asked Teresa.

Joe and Maria laughed. "No, nothing like that. Besides, I would need your help to raise another child and you'll be off at college!"

Now the girls laughed too. "Thank goodness," they said. "That's another incentive for going to college!"

"No homework tonight. I'm getting to bed early. This has been a very tiring week," said Victoria, and the party broke up.

Joe and Maria decided to put off the rest of their research project for the rest of the evening as they had already made much progress.

"My head is swimming with all the information anyway," said Maria. "Vicki was right. This has been a tiring week."

Joe agreed. "Anyway, the Internet will be there tomorrow."

Joe poured them each a glass of wine and they sat in the living room, not really watching the news. Not much was going on in the world, but the weatherman made his report, indicating that the weather for the weekend was to be ideal.

"It looks like Spring may be early," commented Maria.

"Don't count on it too much," laughed Joe. "You know what that will do."

"Yes. 'The best laid plans of mice and men…'"

Maria proposed that they call Bill and Rosario and suggest that they go ahead with the picnic they had been discussing. "It looks like the nice weather will continue through this weekend. Perhaps we could have it tomorrow during the middle of the day when it will be warm."

"That's a great idea," said Joe looking at his watch. "Bill and Rosario are surely still up. They seldom go to bed before midnight on weekends."

They made the call and the suggestion was received warmly. Planning the outing, Maria and Rosario agreed to not try to coordinate menus, but that each family would bring enough for themselves, then they would all share.

Joe felt good again when they went to bed, and said to himself "This is going to work out."

On Saturday morning they told the girls about the picnic plan. Both were excited by the prospect.

They made a list of what they would need and Joe went to the store.

They called Rosario and Bill again in the morning to plan the meeting location and time. They all agreed to go to the Reserva Ecológica Costanera Sur, a big park near the Rio de la Plata. Although it was the middle of the winter according to the calendar, the day was mild and the crowds consequently were large. While the adults set up the portable table and chairs and put out the food, the girls and Billy went for a short walk on the Boardwalk and watched birds and wildlife in the natural setting of the ecological reserve.

After they ate, the younger generation left to do more exploring, while the adults sat and discussed life. Eventually, Rosario and Maria got into a discussion of the tournament and what might be suggested for the next year's event. They had both been recognized as being important contributors and had been appointed to the planning committee.

In the meantime, Bill and Joe sat to one side and Joe filled Bill in on what had happened with the doctor on Friday and the research he had done since that time. Bill reported that he had talked to Dennis, and that his situation hadn't changed.

Joe said he would keep Bill up to speed on his own progress and would be happy to do whatever he could to help with Dennis.

"One thing I have figured out is that by working actively to find an answer I have been able to maintain a high degree of hope, and this seems to more than counteract the despair that I sometimes have that things might not work out. I also have noticed that my focus is less on work and material things, and much more on my family and the good things of life. This cancer is a game-changer in terms of how a person would view life. In some ways it's like the bubble has burst. I notice that I have sheltered myself in the past about others who are battling cancer. In retrospect I wish I had paid more attention to cancer and its impact on so many. Humility and empathy sets in."

Bill nodded. "I can understand that. It's apparent that your approach is a decided contrast with what I observed when I spent those two days with Dennis and Barbara. It has resulted in a very different outlook on your part."

They had come to picnic in the middle of the day. While it was a beautiful day, it was still winter and the sun would be setting early. So they gathered up their possessions and left for home. Joe told Bill he would keep him up to date on his research progress, and Bill agreed to let Joe know if he heard anything from Dennis.

Joe and Maria decided to wait until the next day to resume their research. They were concerned that if they pushed too hard they might get sloppy and miss something important.

They read the paper and had a little wine and listened to their favorite radio station, then went to bed early. The girls got their weekend homework finished and turned in early, too.

Joe woke up in the middle of the night. This was happening more frequently. The house was quiet. Maria was breathing evenly as she slept beside him. He got up as quietly as he could and went to the bathroom. Then he slipped down the hall and listened at the door to the girls' room. He could hear them breathing. He slipped back into bed and lay there, worrying. He had faith that things were going to work out, but he would sure prefer if this episode had already passed and he knew that they were over it. The fears and worries were a big burden. What if the doctors were wrong and the cancer had progressed farther than they realized? What if he couldn't identify a type of treatment that would resolve the problem or left him facing adverse effects for the rest of his life? What if the treatment didn't work? What would become of Maria and the girls if he died? He lay awake for a long time thinking these and other similar thoughts. Finally, he went to sleep and dreamed that he was a boy playing baseball with the kids in the neighborhood. Every time it came to be his turn to bat, the kids would skip him and pass his turn to the next batter. He would ask what was going on, but no one would speak to him.

When he got up, he decided not to talk to Maria right away about his worrying or about his odd dream, but to confide some of his concerns to her at a later time. He was tired and still somewhat worried. He took a shower, shaved, and dressed, which made him feel much better. He went into the kitchen where Maria had made a fresh pot of coffee, and the aroma further improved his mood.

After breakfast, the girls went to a nearby park to play tennis. Joe and Maria took their coffee into the home office and resumed their research.

"Okay. We have identified all of the practical solutions to the problem of what therapies are available. Now we need to go through each and determine the plusses and minuses and begin to narrow the list to what is best in my situation."

"Yes, practical solutions. How come we can't just get Harry Potter's wand when we need it?"

Joe agreed, laughing.

They reviewed their list.

"To start with," suggested Maria, "let's eliminate the ones that won't do and see what's left."

"Good idea, but let me suggest a slightly different approach. Let's eliminate the ones that are not indicated, and put the others into two categories: the ones that appear to be undesirable and the ones that are not. This way we won't eliminate something that we might have to go back to."

"Okay," said Maria. "Let's put plusses and minuses by each of the items in the last two groups."

"Good," said Joe.

They went through the list, checking their notes and some of their web sources as they went. After they finished what Joe referred to as the first cut review, their reworked whiteboard looked like this:

possibilities:

- proton beam therapy - PLUS: adverse impacts relatively minimal compared to other treatments; MINUS: more expensive/not widely available
- radiation (x-ray) - PLUS: widely available/no surgery; MINUS: impacts adjacent tissue, as well as entry and exit damage/possible recurrence of cancer as a side effect
- radiation (Cyberknife) - PLUS: may be more accurate than x-ray/no surgery; MINUS: still impacts adjacent tissue as well as entry and exit/still possibility of producing other cancers/no data yet on side effects/not widely available in South America
- brachytherapy (internal radiation) - PLUS: widely available/less impact than external x-ray or surgery; MINUS: may cause ED/concern: safety of others (from radiation)

not preferred:

- surgery (radical, etc.) - PLUS: widely available/no radiation (although may be needed after); MINUS: damage to other tissues/possible recurrence of cancer/may not get all cancer

- chemotherapy - suppresses immune system/not highly effective - more indicated for advanced cancers
- hormone therapy - reduce or eliminate testosterone/indicated for advanced cancers/does not resolve cancer, just limits its expansion

not indicated:

- "watchful waiting" - allows cancer to continue to grow
- cryosurgery - "freezes" cancer/high risk of impotence
- biologic therapy - bolsters immune system - little information
- high intensity focused ultrasound (HIFU) - "cooks" cancer (approved in some countries/not in US)/ultrasound may "bounce"

As they were conducting their analysis, Joe and Maria could see how the pattern was beginning to emerge; they decided to focus their attention more closely on proton therapy.

When they broke for lunch, Joe felt like they were making serious progress. He concluded that it was like they were having an Aha! moment and were nearing the answer.

As they were finishing lunch, Maria got a call from Rosario saying there was a called meeting of the tennis tournament coordinating committee. Maria told Rosario that she was on her way.

While she was gone, Joe resumed his website searches, specifically on proton therapy.

He researched the history of proton beam therapy. He discovered that the use of proton beams as an effective treatment method was made by Robert R. Wilson in a paper published in 1946 while he was involved in the design of the Harvard Cyclotron Laboratory (HCL). The first treatments were performed with particle accelerators built for physics research, notably at the Berkeley Radiation Laboratory and in Sweden in the fifties. In 1961, collaboration began between HCL and the Massachusetts General Hospital to pursue proton therapy. Over the next four decades, this program refined and expanded these techniques while treating over nine thousand patients. The world's first hospital-based proton therapy center was built in 1990 at the Loma Linda University Medical Center in Loma Linda, California, using equipment that had originally been constructed for research purposes.

Joe also researched how proton beam therapy works and how it is different from other forms of external radiation.

He found out that unlike x-rays (which were classified as photon), protons have a unique characteristic known as the "Bragg peak." X-rays go directly through the body with only a small loss of energy as they pass through flesh and bones. By doing this, they damage normal, healthy cells on their way to the target tumor and beyond. By contrast, the proton beam travels to a point (the Bragg peak) where almost all its energy is delivered, after which it fades. Because of this, the beam will travel harmlessly through the body to the tumor, build up and deliver its energy, and then fade. The technician in control of the machine sets the beam so that the Bragg peak will occur at the site of the tumor. In addition, the beam can be shaped to conform to the shape of the tumor.

Joe found a paper produced by a doctor at the University of Pennsylvania that compared statistics on adverse side effects for various forms of treatment. The paper showed that proton beam patients experienced considerably lower overall adverse side effects of treatment as compared with patient's undergoing other forms. Joe reasoned that this was in large part due to the ability to aim the beam more precisely at the tumor and avoid impacting other tissue.

Joe recalled that the urologist had described surgery as the gold standard, and wondered why proton beam therapy wasn't regarded as the gold standard. It appeared to have many advantages over surgery and even x-ray radiation. He now understood the quote he read to "go with proton, not photon."

Joe was becoming excited that he might be on to something.

After studying proton beam therapy extensively, Joe shifted his approach. Now he didn't focus on websites posted by hospitals and government cancer institutions, but on blogs and similar individual postings. This latter set of resources was generally reflective of information from non-medical individuals who had suffered or were suffering from prostate cancer and were seeking or had completed treatment using proton beam therapy. As such, their stories were not the result of elaborate scientific research studies but were personal accounts that were in many ways more meaningful to Joe. By and large, the blog posts consistently told a story of individuals who were fearful when they encountered the disease, sought answers and assurance, found answers more from others like themselves than from the official medical community, and were very clear about their experience with their treatment.

Joe observed that the men writing these blogs were a different breed from the men who blindly took the information given to them by their doctors. Those men generally did not pursue answers to their questions but simply accepted the information from the doctors.

In his research Joe also came across blogs and articles from people he classified as naysayers. He knew from reading articles and blogs by former proton beam prostate patients that many objections came from the doctors. In some cases, this was because the doctor was an advocate of the form of treatment he provided. Surgeons tended to advocate surgery while radiation oncologists tended to favor radiation therapy. Joe decided that he should expect to run into these naysayers from time to time and he would need to be able to deal with their arguments.

Joe's uncle had been a salesman. He had always told Joe that everyone has to be a salesman. "You might not be selling cars or refrigerators," he used to say, "but you may be selling yourself and your ideas. The techniques are all the same."

One technique he taught Joe was the need to address the buyer's objections. "Don't try to address each objection as it comes up. Wait and get the buyer to list all of his objections. Then, and only then, after he has given you all of his objections, should you address them. Then when you do, go through the points logically and succinctly, one at a time. This way, the momentum of the discussion will be in your favor and you will be controlling the conversation. Assuming you know your product and its benefits, you will be able to counter all his points. During the process respond to one of his points and get him to agree that what you say is correct. After he agrees on that point, move to the next. He may not buy your product but he will be a lot closer than he would have been if you had not organized the conversation. Prepare for this by knowing your product and really knowing its properties. Also try to think of all the possible objections and when you hear a new one add it to your inventory and develop one or more responses to each objection. You'll be a good salesman. I can tell."

Based on his uncle's advice, Joe decided to prepare for the objections. Joe knew from his research that not everyone was convinced of the benefits of proton beam therapy. Joe made a summary of the objections he had encountered, along with possible responses, as follows:

Some cancers cannot be treated by proton therapy and there are some situations where proton is inappropriate. This included situations where the cancer had not been treated early enough and had metastasized. The principal characteristic of proton therapy is the ability to target a specific location and bombard it with a higher dosage. For a cancer that occurs in several locations, or for a cancer that has spread, the proton beam would not by its nature be effective. In these cases, hormone and chemotherapy were more likely indicated. These cases also sometimes called for more traditional radiation even though it would result in greater damage to healthy tissue.

Proton therapy is too expensive compared to other treatments. Proton treatment is more expensive partly because the equipment required is enormously expensive, particularly the cyclotron and the gantry systems. The first installations cost $200 or $300 million. Refinements in design have brought the cost down to closer to $130 million, and the prospect is for further reductions in the future. In addition, development is underway for designs for smaller centers that can be successful in more rural areas. Just because it is new and still in development does not mean that it is undesirable as a form of therapy. The cost to the patient for treatment of prostate cancer at a center in the United States might be around $150,000 to $180,000, while the cost of treatment in Korea, for example, may be closer to a third of that figure. Either way, consideration should be given to the total cost of addressing the disease over the patient's lifetime, not just the cost of the principal form of treatment.

Because of the reduced side effects of proton beam treatment, the cost over a lifetime of treatment can be closer to (or even less) than the cost of other forms of treatment. For example, traditional x-ray radiation or brachytherapy may result in the development of secondary cancers that then need to be treated. Similarly, surgery may fail to remove all the cancer and may in turn require radiation or even proton beam therapy. Even "watchful waiting" requires long term monitoring, including additional testing (such as biopsies) and possibly a lifetime of drug and hormone therapy.

Also, there has to be consideration of the cost of side effects. Men who are treated with surgery or traditional radiation are much more likely to experience impotence, erectile dysfunction, and loss of bladder control or leakage. These may not be costs in a monetary sense, but these are very much costs to the individual and his spouse and their enjoyment of life.

Finally, Joe observed that the higher cost was largely attributable to the fact that this is relatively new technology. Joe knew from his own experience in engineering that innovation in design, construction, and operational procedures would bring the overall cost down over time.

Proton therapy is experimental or unproven. This objection stems from the relatively recent and rapid evolution of proton beam therapy. Surgery dates from the end of the 19th century, and x-ray radiation dates almost back to the discovery of x-rays in 1895. While proton beam therapy was conceived in the middle of the 20th century, the equipment and the control systems (computers) needed to make it work were not sophisticated enough until the 1990s. Since then, only eleven treatment centers have been developed - nine in the United States and one each in Korea and Germany. Data is still being collected to evaluate proton in comparison to other forms of treatment but studies are being released that demonstrate the effectiveness of proton and the significantly lower level of adverse effects.

Joe knew that many of the official websites were reluctant to conclude formally that proton therapy was better than other forms of treatment. Indeed, while proton beam therapy has been in use for several decades, the scientific studies on long-term effectiveness were just starting to become available.

Apart from empirical studies, there are many advocates of proton who suggest that the greater accuracy and the ability to deliver higher doses to cancer cells with less impact on nearby healthy tissue makes this form of treatment inherently more desirable. The fact that there are significantly fewer and less severe side effects contributes to that conclusion. This sounded pretty logical to Joe.

More time and further studies will reveal whether there is any difference between proton beam therapy and other forms of treatment in the degree of recurrence over the long term, and the emergence of long-term side effects.

Not more effective than other treatments. From his reading, Joe observed that this objection is another way of articulating the other objections. In other words, if proton beam therapy is not better than the other therapies, is it worth the additional cost? And how can it be shown to be better if there are no studies showing that fewer men die or that men live longer compared to the other treatments?

One difficulty was that, compared with the number of individuals who have been treated by other means, only a small number of patients have been treated by proton therapy. This was changing, however. Around 30,000 patients had been treated for prostate cancer at the oldest hospital-based facility (Loma Linda University Medical Center in California, USA) since 1990, and follow-up studies were beginning to indicate positive results, at least as good as for other forms of treatment. In addition, in Joe's mind the significantly reduced side effects made this form of treatment more desirable.

Joe concluding his review of the negative arguments, and decided to return to Amazon to take another look at books. He finally ordered two more books for express shipping. These books specifically discussed proton therapy.

Just as he completed his Amazon order, Maria returned from the tournament committee meeting. Joe showed her the results of his research and analysis. He also showed her information on the books he had ordered from Amazon.

"The interesting thing about looking at the books," he explained, "was that when I was looking at books about surgery, several of them had to do with overcoming the side effects of surgery, not on any advantages of surgery itself. The other forms of treatment didn't list books of that type."

"I'm pretty convinced," said Maria when Joe had finished. "Looks like now we'll only have to deal with the cost issue and see if there is a center that can take you."

"That will be our topic for tomorrow. For now, however, I'm bushed and need to let my mind rest."

"Good deal," said Maria.

Websites Joe and Maria used to identify and evaluate treatment options

Note: for updated information on websites and other information in this book, please see www.RoadToNamiIsland.blogspot.com.

http://www.mayoclinic.com/health/prostate-cancer/DS00043/DSECTION=treatments-and-drugs

http://www.cancer.org/Cancer/ProstateCancer/DetailedGuide/prostate-cancer-treating-considering-options

http://prostateprotontherapy.blogspot.com/p/prostate-cancer-treatment-options.html

http://www.protonbob.com/proton-treatment-homepage.asp

http://www.prostate-cancer-institute.com/

http://www.mdanderson.org/patient-and-cancer-information/cancer-information/cancer-types/prostate-cancer/index.html

http://www.cancer.org/cancer/prostatecancer/detailedguide/prostate-cancer-treating-considering-options

http://familydoctor.org/online/famdocen/home/common/cancer/treatment/264.html

http://prostateprotontherapy.blogspot.com/2010/04/prostate-cancer-treatment-options.html

http://knol.google.com/k/curtis-poling/prostate-cancer-treatment-compilation/3ud6fqyg50117/2#

http://www.webmd.com/prostate-cancer/guide/prostate-cancer-treatments

http://www.cdc.gov/cancer/prostate/basic_info/treatment.htm

http://en.wikipedia.org/wiki/Radiation_therapy

http://www.prostate-cancer.org/education/localdis/brosman_RP2003.html

http://en.wikipedia.org/wiki/Bragg_peak

http://en.wikipedia.org/wiki/Proton_therapy

http://protoninfo.com/Articles/UniversityofPennsylvania.pdf

http://exsitewebware.com/extrema/bragg.html

Relevant articles at Wikipedia:

"prostate cancer"

"management of prostate cancer"

"proton beam therapy"

Websites with information about diagnosis and analysis of prostate cancers

http://en.wikipedia.org/wiki/Prostate_biopsy

http://en.wikipedia.org/wiki/Gleason_score

http://www.cancer.org/Cancer/ProstateCancer/DetailedGuide/prostate-cancer-staging

http://www.phoenix5.org/Infolink/ClinicalStaging.html

Websites and blogs with information from patients

http://affordableprotontherapy.blogspot.com/

http://www.yananow.org/

http://protondon.blogspot.com/

http://health.groups.yahoo.com/group/protoninfo/messages

Books on prostate cancer and treatment options

[Note: if you look through books on the Amazon website, one useful technique is to review the reader comments for each book, including both the favorable and "most helpful negative comments." The unfavorable ones give you an idea of whether the information is useful and whether the book represents any particular biases.]

"You Can Beat Prostate Cancer: And You Don't Need Surgery to Do It" by Robert J. Marckini

"Prostate Cancer Meets The Proton Beam: A Patient's Experience" by Fuller Jones

"Don't Fear the Big Dogs" by Bill Vancil

CHAPTER 4. PROTON

On Monday morning, with the girls off to school and Maria off to the school library, Joe decided to take care of some things at his office and then return home to continue his research. On his way to work he mentally planned his morning activities. He decided that unless there was an emergency of some kind, he would finish up and then go home to focus on his prostate cancer research. When he got to the office there were only a few messages from Friday and none were critical. He expected that would be the case since his assistant would have called him to let him know about anything that was significant. He returned the calls fairly quickly and took care of some letters and other tasks.

Then he turned his attention to his principal interest of the moment.

He placed two phone calls. The first was to his urologist. He asked the receptionist if there would be an opportunity for him and Maria to come in and see the doctor in the next few days, as they were coming to a decision on a course of treatment and wanted to confer with the urologist. This would be for a consultation, not a full exam.

"Yes you may," the receptionist said, "but the first opportunity will be this Thursday."

After making the appointment he placed the next call to his health insurance company. Joe had not had many dealings with the company and did not know exactly what the proper procedure would be.

When he was connected with a representative, he gave her his name and account number and proceeded to describe his situation.

"I have been diagnosed with prostate cancer and it has been recommended to me by my urologist that I undergo surgery to remove the prostate. I have done some research and concluded that I would prefer not to take that advice, but to undergo what is called proton beam therapy. I have learned that this type of treatment is not available in Argentina, but is an approved treatment and is available in other countries. I need to find out what my plan will cover if I proceed in this direction."

As a non-citizen, Joe was not eligible for the country's health care system other than for emergency care. Argentine citizens (including Maria and the girls) were eligible for services provided by the government and could also belong to plans offered by trade and professional organizations. They and non-citizens alike were also eligible for private insurance plans. When he left the contractor to start his own consulting organization, Joe had elected to get a very basic policy with an eye on building up his business before he upgraded.

The representative indicated that they had a fairly straightforward procedure for handling this type of claim.

"Generally, we don't pay for services received outside of the country. But if your doctor, in this case probably the urologist, writes us a letter and states that the procedure is medically necessary and is not available within Argentina, we will pay for a portion of the cost. We will also pay for a portion of services provided in this country, such as diagnostic services. In all cases you will pay a percentage and we will pay a percentage."

She advised Joe that the policy had a cap on the total and that the insurance company would pay for a total equivalent of about $25,000 in US dollars.

Finally, she let Joe know that any amount spent outside of the country would be in the form of a reimbursement. Joe would have to pay the bill and then submit for reimbursement for the insurance company's portion.

Joe thanked the representative and got her name and the phone number of her direct line so he could call her if he had any other questions. She also agreed to send Joe the forms he would need to request the reimbursement, along with information about getting the sign-off from the doctor.

Joe sat back and reviewed where he was and what his next steps would be. He had determined that proton beam therapy (or PBT) was his choice for treatment. He and Maria had been through most of the research together and were pretty much of a like mind on everything, but the actual decision had only been forming in his mind since Sunday afternoon while Maria was at the tennis tournament meeting. They had only been able to talk about it for a short time. He decided that his first step would be to confirm that Maria was in full agreement.

The next step would be to confer with the urologist on Thursday and get the doctor's input. He didn't know if he would face objections there or not, but he had already started the process of identifying possible objections and preparing to answer them. While he expected that the urologist would not be completely happy with Joe's rejection of his recommendation, he didn't expect there to be a major fuss.

In the meantime he would focus on gathering information for the next step, which would be to determine which facility would be the best to use for his treatment. Perhaps he could have an answer before Thursday and would be able to use the information in his discussions with the urologist.

"Okay," he thought to himself. "Now I have a plan. Time to act."

At lunch time, he collected his thumb drive and paperwork, then took the bus home.

When Joe got home he went directly to the home office, grabbing a sandwich on the way. He carefully copied everything on the whiteboard to a pad of paper, then erased it to start a new list.

Proton Beam Therapy Facilities

- locate facilities
- establish criteria
- match facilities to criteria

Joe looked at his list. It looked easy. Joe knew, however, that when something looks easy it often isn't.

Joe then went to the Internet and began his research. He went to Google and Yahoo, typing in key words such as proton therapy, prostate cancer treatment proton therapy, etc. Each time he found a lead he followed it and made a note on the whiteboard.

Soon Joe found the website for the National Association for Proton Therapy. Here he found links to various proton centers operating worldwide, including those already in existence, as well as those that are under construction or under development. By checking several of the links, Joe brought the list up to date.

Joe reasoned that the ones under development or construction would not help. This left him with nine operational centers in the United States and two others. One of these was in Germany and one was in Korea.

Joe went to the website for each of the eleven centers and made notes, being sure to copy the site addresses so he could show all the information to Maria.

Before long, the girls arrived home, followed by Maria.

Even though Joe had been home all afternoon, he had not given any thought to cooking. Usually when he was working alone at home he would put a roast in the oven, pull something out of the freezer to defrost, or make some other move toward getting dinner ready. But today he had been very much occupied with his task.

"Not to worry," said Maria putting away her coat. "We have lots of leftovers from the picnic and they need to be used."

Everyone enjoyed the leftovers, which had been combined and then divided up by the two families. The result was that they had a little bit of many different things.

After supper and the obligatory recitation of the interesting happenings for the day, the girls went off to do homework. Joe and Maria sat down in the home office with coffee. Joe proceeded to bring Maria up to date on the upcoming appointment with the urologist and on his phone conversation with the insurance company representative.

Maria agreed that she could be available for the appointment with the urologist, but she frowned when it came to discussing the cost of treatment.

"How can we afford to pursue this treatment?" she asked.

Joe was ready. "I look at it more as how can we afford not to? I'm in my mid-fifties. I have twenty or thirty good years left in me and I want to be here for you and the girls as long as I can. I also want to be useful to you. I don't want to be constantly having to deal with complications or side effects of the various forms of treatment. From what I can tell, treatment of some of these side effects can actually cost some serious money, so if a treatment is cheaper initially, it may not be in the long run. This is a lot like what I do in engineering, where we consider the life-cycle cost: that is, the cost of a solution over the entire lifespan of the project, including operation and maintenance, rather than just the cost of the initial construction.

"I suggest," he continued "that we focus some additional research on what facilities can provide this service and what their costs would be. If we can't make it work, we'll drop back to the next best plan and see what we can do there."

Maria thought a minute and said "You make a persuasive argument. I do want you in one piece, and I really don't want this hanging over us for years. Let's see what we can do."

"I have also summarized what we have done to date, so that we can discuss the options with the urologist on Thursday. I'm not expecting a significant negative reaction, but my father always told me to be prepared."

He proceeded to run through their research over the last few days and their conclusions.

Maria was impressed. "You've been busy. This puts it a little more in an organized thought process," she said.

Joe reviewed the list of existing proton facilities.

"There are a number of other proton facilities around the world, but these are mostly equipped for research and are not designed to handle human patients."

The results of his research indicated the following possibilities:

- James M. Slater, M.D. Proton Treatment and Research Center at Loma Linda University Medical Center, Loma Linda, California (USA)
- The University of Florida Proton Therapy Institute, Shands Hospital, Jacksonville, Florida (USA)
- The University of Texas M.D. Anderson Cancer Center's Proton Center, Houston, Texas (USA)

- ProCure Proton Therapy Center, located at the INTEGRIS Cancer Campus, Oklahoma City, Oklahoma (USA)
- CDH Proton Center/ProCure Proton Therapy Center, near Naperville, Illinois (Suburban Chicago, USA)
- The Roberts Proton Therapy Center at University of Pennsylvania Health System, Philadelphia, Pennsylvania (USA)
- Hampton University Proton Therapy Institute, Hampton, Virginia (USA)
- Francis H. Burr Proton Therapy Center, Massachusetts General Hospital, Boston, Massachusetts (USA)
- Indiana University Health Proton Therapy Center, Bloomington, Indiana (USA)
- Rinecker Proton Therapy Center, Munich, Germany
- National Cancer Center/Proton Beam Therapy Center Korea, Seoul, South Korea

Now that Joe and Maria had developed a list of possible sources for treatment, the next step was to evaluate the choices and make a decision. As the result of his background in engineering, this was the kind of logical process with which Joe was very familiar.

They first made a list of what should be the criteria for making a decision. The list they came up with included (in no particular order):

Accessibility - At first they said location, but changed that since (unless the facility was in Buenos Aires) where it was located was less important than the ability to get to it easily and find a place to stay.

Delay - How quickly could Joe start getting treatment? This was a key. Joe had learned that while about two-thirds of prostate cancers grow slowly, the rest do not. In some cases, the longer it takes to get treatment can have an effect on the chances for success.

Qualifications - How experienced the staff and doctors were in providing this particular treatment, and how good was the overall quality of care.

Advancement in Treatment - Whether the facility was keeping up with advances in the state of the art. Maria suggested this one, reasoning that if there was a rapid advance in techniques or technology, a facility would need to evaluate those advances and incorporate the appropriate ones into the treatment programs. This criterion suggested that extra credit go to facilities that are linked to a research hospital or an institution that conducts studies aimed at improving care.

Cost - As Joe was covered by an insurance plan that would only partially reimburse him for treatment, he needed to be sure that he could afford it.

Intangibles - Joe studied the list. His uncle was a salesman and had always preached "price, product, and service" as being the principal elements in making a buying decision. Joe thought about this, and suggested adding this one more criterion. Since he would necessarily have to travel to a strange and distant place to undergo treatment, Joe was concerned that he not be required to spend a lot of time in a place with few amenities. He felt that the success of his treatment would be affected by whether or not his time was spent having a good time versus being left to mope around being homesick.

Joe and Maria divided the list of proton centers and tackled each criterion in order and compared their findings. At each stage, they marked individual facilities either up or down based on this research.

At the end of the process, their consensus was that the ideal facility for obtaining treatment would be the National Cancer Center (NCC) in Seoul, Korea.

Their reasoning went as follows:

Accessibility - There was no facility in Argentina, or, for that matter, in South America. Consequently, all of the facilities were in locations where Joe would have to go and stay for an extended period. In this respect they were all equally accessible from Buenos Aires. The facilities all appeared to have adequate temporary housing for those away from home, although one or two appeared to be more convenient for people in the immediate area who would likely be using the facility on an out-patient basis. The NCC stood out since the program actually included housing as part of arrangements and was in an area with excellent public transportation. It looked to Joe as if spending a number of weeks in Seoul would not involve giving up any mobility. As a bonus, Joe and Maria surmised that, the fact that because the patients were being housed near each other, there was more of a chance for mutual support and information exchange.

Delay - The NCC won hands down here, since treatment could begin in as little as two weeks. Other facilities had waiting lists of up to two or three months.

Qualifications - Several of the facilities were associated with medical schools at institutions of higher learning, but the NCC stood out as being an all-encompassing facility, with research and training functions along with treatment. The NCC was a major player in the Korean national strategy for addressing cancer, assisting in developing and maintaining the country's cancer policy, and working with cancer treatments at regional and local levels, not just nationally. The NCC took a comprehensive approach, including diagnosis, treatment, follow-up treatment and care, and overall health care.

Advancements in Treatment - As with a couple of the other facilities, NCC conducts research, makes studies to advance the state of the art, and trains in-service professionals of all types in understanding and utilizing new techniques.

Cost - Here again, NCC in Korea was the winner. If Joe was located in the United States, had a health insurance plan that covered the service, or was an elderly or poor person, he might be able to obtain treatment at little or no direct cost to himself. Otherwise, treatment in the United States generally costs two to three times the cost of treatment in Korea. In addition, the plans at most facilities included the treatment and related medical services, but did not include housing. At eight or nine weeks, the housing expense could become significant.

Finally, the "Intangible Element" - While each of the facilities was located in areas where there would be much to do, Korea was obviously a new and exciting place that would keep Joe occupied and make the time go more quickly. Joe had traveled back and forth to the United States many times and had traveled extensively throughout South America. Other than one brief trip to Saudi Arabia many years ago on behalf of the contractor, he had not been anywhere else in the world. He thought about Teresa's school project on Korea and decided he needed to look again at her report.

After narrowing the field to the National Cancer Center in Korea, Joe and Maria did additional exploring to find out what they could about the institution itself, as well as the community and nation in which it is located.

On the whiteboard, Joe made a list:

- healthy and interesting cuisine
- healthy environment
- modern technology
- advanced society mixed with ancient culture
- home to the 2018 Winter Olympics

Joe and Maria spent the better part of Monday and Tuesday evenings getting the information assembled and analyzed. Tuesday evening, Joe found a website with information on how to contact the NCC, which was done through a representative in the United States. Joe recognized the name Curtis Poling from several of the searches he had done over the past few weeks. As a prostate cancer patient, Mr. Poling had been treated at Loma Linda in California. Afterwards he took up the task of helping other men get information on the option of proton beam therapy for prostate cancer and had been enlisted by KMI, the company that handles marketing for the NCC, to help bring patients to Korea.

On Wednesday, Maria attended a meeting of the tournament planning committee with Rosario while Joe stayed home to make notes and practice his presentation for the urologist. He went over his notes with Maria when she returned.

After they were finished, they both agreed that they were happy with the result. Joe felt good and felt prepared for the discussion with the urologist scheduled for the next day.

On Thursday they had breakfast with the girls. Soon after the girls left for school Joe and Maria drove to the urologist's office.

The urologist smiled when Joe came in. "So, how did the research project go? Are you ready to choose surgery?" he asked.

"It went very well. And like you guessed, the decision process is much like one would use to solve an engineering problem." They both chuckled.

Joe related how he and his wife had conducted the research and evaluated the information at each step of the process, including the criteria they use to develop the decision and how the criteria applied to each of the choices they had evaluated.

"In summary," Joe concluded, "We have decided that I should seek proton beam treatment at the National Cancer Center in Seoul, Korea. The NCC offers the most immediate availability and the most reasonable cost. It is a top-quality facility which reflects research, along with clinical application of the knowledge. I am confident that if I can be accepted I will be satisfied with the outcome."

"That's really impressive," said the doctor. "I have never seen a patient spend so much time and energy making such a careful study to determine his choices. Although I have to tell you that I am a little surprised by the outcome. I have attended many seminars and courses to keep up my professional skills and knowledge and have yet to hear this much about proton therapy. Perhaps you could give me a synopsis of what it is and why it is preferable."

Joe detected that this was a little bit of a trick question and the doctor was testing whether Joe really knew what he was talking about. He had noticed that even in the professional sounding articles he had read online it sounded like some doctors refused to consider choices that were obviously available. He had also noticed that the individuals who wrote blogs telling of their experiences often had to argue with doctors, some even going for second and third opinions before they found a doctor who legitimately considered the proton option. As Joe understood it this stemmed, in part, from the fact that many doctors had vested interests in certain treatments, such as surgeons who advocated surgery, or radiation oncologists who supported radiation.

It occurred to Joe that his salesman uncle might describe it as being like the Chevrolet salesman sending a customer down the street to the Ford dealer.

But to be perfectly fair, it might be due to the fact that proton therapy was not even available in South America and that few could, as a practical matter, elect this option.

Joe proceeded to give a general, layman's explanation of proton beam therapy. Joe and Maria were silently glad Joe had done his homework.

"Tell me about what you concluded about the cost consideration," the urologist asked.

Again, Joe detected that the doctor was looking for a chink in Joe's conclusions and resolve to pursue proton therapy. He was glad to find out that the doctor was asking the same questions he and Maria had already asked themselves and had answered.

"Well again, I approached it from the point of view of an engineer. In engineering, we deal often with what we call 'life-cycle cost.' This refers to the cost of a facility as not being just the cost of constructing it but the cost of construction, operation, maintenance, etc., over its entire useful life. So when we compare several different design concepts for a project, we consider all these factors together. In my case I took into account the cost of the treatment, which is higher than some of the other treatment choices, but I also took into account the possible need for follow-up treatment, as might be necessary with other treatment options that might not get all of the cancer. In those cases, additional treatments, such as radiation or chemotherapy may be needed after the initial treatment. I also took into account the non-financial cost of side effects, such as radiation damage to healthy tissue, incontinence, impotence, and so forth. When I took all these things into account, along with the fact that I have a good many more years of life I want to live, I decided there is really no option."

The doctor nodded gravely, and then broke into a grin. "I guess I should have expected that you would come up with an engineering solution to that problem too," he exclaimed. "I believe you are committed to this course of treatment. I can't help you much more than you have already helped yourself. I can't provide the treatment you are seeking. After you have completed it, I will be happy to continue to do your follow-up monitoring here. What can I do for you next?"

"I have made an initial approach to Mr. Curtis Poling, the representative of the company that handles marketing for the National Cancer Center," said Joe. "His office is in the United States and serves the interests of the NCC outside of Korea. I have submitted a questionnaire to him by email and am to gather some medical information and forward it to him. He will be my point of contact for this process. He will forward the information to the NCC in Seoul and will let me know what other information will be needed. I expect to have an answer from them in a week or so. I will contact you if I need any further information. I will also need a letter from you for my insurance company indicating that the treatment I am seeking is medically necessary."

"OK," said the urologist. "I will have your medical records provided to you in digital form so you can transmit them to the proper parties. Also I will have the letter prepared."

They agreed that Joe would stop by the next morning to get the records and the letter so they could be forwarded.

After Joe and Maria left, they stopped in at an ice cream parlor and had a treat.

"I was somewhat nervous about that meeting," admitted Maria. "I didn't know how he was going to act. I think that once you showed him what you knew, he figured you weren't taking this casually and that he wasn't going to be able to push you into accepting a treatment not of your own choosing."

"Yeah," said Joe, mulling it all over. "The best way to approach this type of situation is to be prepared. If you know your subject and feel good and solid in your positions, people aren't going to be able to push you around. They will only be able to push you around if you let them. And if you're the one doing the pushing and you run into someone who obviously doesn't want to be pushed, you need to give up and move to the next customer where you might fare better."

When he got home, Joe called Doctor Silva's office and asked that his general medical records be provided to him on a CD so he could forward them to the NCC.

These had been a very hectic few days, so supper that evening was ordering pizza again.

"Wow," exclaimed Teresa. "I don't know what's going on, but ordering pizza twice in - what - two or three weeks is amazing!"

After supper, Joe and Maria sat and listened to their favorite radio station while the girls finished homework.

"The next big part of this is to bring the girls into the loop," said Joe. "They need to be told. Anyway, they have been suspicious that something is afoot."

"Agreed," said Maria. "Let's do that sometime this weekend when we have enough time and everyone is not running all around."

"Agreed," said Joe.

Joe picked up the medical information at the offices of the two doctors on Friday morning and took the CD's to his own office so he could transmit the digital files to Mr. Poling in the United States by email. He knew that Mr. Poling would forward them directly, but he realized that it was after close of business on Friday in Korea, and he would have to wait until the next week for any response.

Afterward, he telephoned Mr. Poling and discussed what had been sent and asked if there was anything else he could do for now.

"No, not now," said Mr. Poling. "The time line goes something like this: once the doctors' committee in Seoul gets the materials, they will review them. They will ask for more information if there is anything further that they need. After they have everything they need, they usually make a decision within a few days to a week. Did you tell me you haven't had a CT scan yet?"

"That's correct," replied Joe.

"They might want one to verify that the cancer has not metastasized into your lymph nodes or other areas. You may as well work on scheduling a CT scan but don't actually do it until the doctors in Seoul tell you to. They might not need it. If you are accepted and go to Korea, they will give you those kinds of tests when you get there. Once you are approved, we will get you a contract and a formal price quote. Almost all communications are by email and will come from my office, so make sure you keep an eye on your inbox. As soon as that paperwork is completed, you will be contacted by my office about logistics and dates. Remember, the price includes the treatment, other related medical care that is needed while you are in Korea, eight weeks of accommodations at an extended stay-type hotel or apartment, other health care needs you might have, and some other amenities. It does not include airfare. You pay for that, although we can help make the arrangements. Also, as a new feature, we will help arrange for a driver and car for the duration of your stay for use in traveling from your temporary residence to the NCC for treatments. Some patients find that they are fully comfortable in dealing with the public transportation system in Seoul.

"You will also need to make sure your passport is up to date and contact a Korean embassy or consulate in your area to check on visa requirements. You might start working on that as soon as you can. Finally, if there is anything I can help you with just contact me at any time. I'll ship a packet of information to you right away. The information in the packet will cover many of the questions you might have."

Joe gave Mr. Poling his mailing address, and then started what would turn out to be the first of many lists, sometimes consolidating and rewriting more than two or three lists a day.

- passport/visa - check requirements
- check immunizations
- airline schedules
- clothes? (weather)
- communications between Korea and home
- electric voltage - electrical appliances and electronics

On Saturday morning Maria was scheduled to go with Rosario to a meeting at the tennis club to discuss next year's tournament. Maria told Joe that she wanted to be involved in the tournament planning and needed to go to the meeting so she would be assured of being appointed to a committee that she wanted. Rosario drove by and picked Maria up.

After the meeting, Rosario suggested they go for a coffee and Maria agreed.

When they had gotten their coffees and found a booth, Rosario brought up the prostate cancer issue.

"It hurts me a lot to know that people I know and love and am very close to are hurting and that I can't do anything about it. Bill is fretting about his friend Dennis, but he can't talk to Joe about it too much because Joe has his own problem. I watched you closely at the meeting. We've known each other since we were little girls in school. I can tell that you're not yourself. I know you are a mature, solid person and can handle a lot, but this may be too much. I don't want you to have a breakdown. You have to talk to me about it."

"Well, in part you are right," Maria started slowly. "Joe is a good man and I love him very much, but he is nervous and it makes me nervous. I can't show it too much or he might fall apart emotionally. I've noticed that he sometimes can't sleep at night. He has to get up a lot to go to the bathroom, but sometimes he just lies in bed. I pretend to be asleep so that I don't bother him and hope that he will go back to sleep. But I know that he is awake and that it's because he is worrying. I know that he is concerned about me and the girls, but he is also concerned about himself, too, which is only natural. After all, he is the one who is facing - well, death, to put it bluntly. It really hit him when he heard about Mr. Ruiz at the tennis tournament. He didn't know the man well, but no one expected that he would be dead just like that. And to find out about it only a week before he officially got his diagnosis didn't help.

"Last night Joe got up and went to the bathroom, but he didn't come back. I thought he had gone into the kitchen, maybe for a glass of water, so I went to see if he needed help. I found him sitting in the living room with the curtain open looking out the picture window, staring at the lights of the city. I asked him if he was okay. He told me he couldn't sleep because he was worried. He said he knew intellectually that everything would work out and that he knew he was carefully making the right decisions. But he knew that planning on what to do and getting it done are two separate things. He said he kept thinking about the premise of the movie *Perfect Storm* in which all the factors that could go wrong came together and produced the worst possible result.

"He told me that if anything happened to him, he knew the girls and I would be taken care of. I have many relatives here in Argentina who will make sure we will be okay. But he went on to say that he knew that his disease is serious and that despite everything he might die. He said he found himself wondering if he would live long enough to meet his grandchildren.

"I told him that I love him and have much faith, both in his ability to research and choose the right answer, but also that God will guide us and help us. But you know, Rosario, this is hard on all us. And before it's done, it will be hard on the girls. We need to talk with them and let them know what is happening. This is no picnic, as Joe would say."

The two women sat quietly for a few minutes, sipping their coffee and thinking.

Rosario was the first to speak. "Do you remember when Bill asked me to marry him? You and I had talked beforehand, thinking that this might happen. The things you told me made a lot of sense, and I have always remembered them. You said that if I had a big decision to make, I should break it down into its various parts and work on each of them separately. You asked me if I loved Bill, and if I could see myself being comfortable living with him for a long time after the glow of the honeymoon had worn off. You also asked me if I had faith in my choices. I thought those things through and decided that I was ready more than ever to have Bill as a life partner. In fact, I nearly asked him and suggested that we elope, but I knew it would break Momma's heart if I didn't have a fancy wedding, so I figured I could even put up with the wedding to meet my ultimate objective.

"I'm going to turn this around on you and ask you to break the issue into its parts and tell me how you see each part."

Maria recapped the current situation using the model Rosario had just discussed. "Joe has prostate cancer. He has carefully researched the forms of treatment that are available and has selected proton beam therapy as being the most advanced treatment available and the most likely to meet his needs. He has also researched the places that provide this therapy and has selected an excellent facility in Korea as the place where he wants to get treated. All in all, I have to agree with Joe that intellectually he has done what he needs to do to make a decision. All we have to worry about now is can he be accepted there and can he get to Korea and will the treatments help make him well. Those are big ifs." She smiled and added, "it's a little like one of those American sports guys that Joe keeps quoting: it ain't over 'til it's over."

"Well, it sounds to me like you and Joe have a handle on the problem and the steps to solve it," Rosario said. "I'd say that you are a long way toward implementing a solution. You need to think positively - the glass is half full, not half empty. Oh, and where did the Korea idea come from? I hadn't heard that part."

"Things do seem to move fast, don't they?" said Maria with a chuckle. She proceeded to run quickly through the research of the past few days and Joe's decision to go to the National Cancer Center in Seoul for treatment.

"He's already started the process of sending his medical information for review and hopes to know in about a week."

"Okay," Rosario breathed out. "You and the girls will have to come over for supper a lot while he's gone."

"And you and the Bills will have to come for supper at our house, too."

"I didn't mean to imply that you can't handle cooking when Joe is gone!" They both laughed.

"It makes me feel better talking this out with you." Maria said.

"Doctor Rosario's office is always open to you." They laughed again.

"Well, get me back to my place. I left Joe making lists, and if I'm not careful, he may already be packing."

On Sunday after a lazy morning and a light lunch, Joe and Maria gathered the girls in the living room.

"You may have noticed that things around here haven't been what you would necessarily call normal over the last few weeks," he began.

There was general agreement by the girls. Maria smiled.

"The situation is important, and it's serious, but it's under control, and everything is going to work out okay."

He realized he was fibbing a little, but he was confident and felt he was going to be able to get what he needed.

"I have a form of cancer known as prostate cancer, which is cancer in a gland near my bladder. It's one of the most common types of cancer men get, just like breast cancer is a significant cancer typically afflicting women. My case is in its very early stages, and it appears that my prognosis for resolving this issue is very good."

The girls were watching him very carefully now, with serious expressions on their faces. He really loved them.

"This type of cancer is typically very slow growing, but I am considered young and it will eventually cause me problems. There are several methods for dealing with this type of cancer, but it can be dealt with effectively if it is done early. Mom and I have done a lot of research and have found the type of treatment that we think would be best. I am now in the process of applying for this type of treatment and hope to know within a week or so whether or not I have been accepted. If all works out well, I will be away from home for a couple of months to get the treatment, but once I have done that, I should have no more cancer problems."

Joe's presentation was short and to the point, but it gave the girls all they needed in order to get the big picture. Joe and Maria had agreed when the girls were born that they would be treated as their maturity warranted, and that they would be kept informed about important family matters. Joe felt that his monologue was at the level it needed to be.

"Now, are there any questions?"

"At least it's not a baby," said Teresa. "We don't have enough room."

"Young? You're considered to be young?" asked Victoria.

Everyone smiled. Joe was concerned that he had not made the case serious enough.

"Now there are many things that can go wrong still, but I believe we have done what we can to mitigate any problems. Mom and I approached this like an engineering problem that requires a carefully analyzed solution."

Everyone agreed that they would ask questions if they had them, and not get worried. Joe and Maria promised to stop anything they were doing and help answer questions or help deal with any concerns that the girls might have.

After the discussion, the girls decided to go for a walk to the park, and Maria ran out to pick up some items for supper. Joe went into the home office and sat down. He was depressed, and before he realized it, a tear came to his eye. He was tired. The pace of work and the emotional pressure from the anxiety of dealing with the prostate cancer was getting to him. The light manner in which the girls treated his announcement hadn't helped.

Intellectually, he knew that he was taking the right approach; actually the only approach he could take. He was approaching the problem like an engineering problem and applying engineering problem-solving methods. But this was not about pouring concrete or fixing a drainage canal or a bridge. This was about him and his body and his mortality. And it was also about his family and the possible consequences on all of them if anything should happen.

He knew that if he didn't, as the British say, "keep a stiff upper lip" the whole family might become emotionally stressed. He needed to keep his wits about him and maintain a solid front to help Maria and the girls get through this. And their ability to get through it would affect his ability to get through it as well.

Since he had been to the urologist a couple of weeks before to find out the results of the biopsy, Joe had told only a few people of his cancer. His intention was not to garner sympathy, but to let them know that he might be unavailable for a time while he was getting treatment. This became even more important as it became more apparent that he would be pursuing proton therapy. He explained to them that this treatment was unavailable locally and would require him to be away for an extended period of time.

Some of the reactions he got from the people he told were a little surprising, and they sometimes tended to make him angry.

People would say "Oh, I know someone who had cancer, and they had it worse than you." Or "You'll be fine. You just have to have the right attitude and you can beat it." Or "Let me tell you about the back operation I had for my slipped disk."

His favorite line was "Oh, please let me know if there is anything I can do for you." As if the person actually had any clue as to what he could do or had any real intention of doing anything at all.

Some of his friends acted like they might catch the cancer from him and avoided him. That had really surprised him, because it made no intellectual sense.

After sitting and thinking about these instances for a while, Joe sighed. He realized that these were probably natural reactions, and that most people wanted to be sympathetic but didn't know how. Joe knew to forgive them and promised himself that when he got through this ordeal (not if he got through it, for he was convinced that he would) he would be very careful how he would treat a sick friend.

About that time, Maria returned from her errand. He went out to greet her and suggested that they sit with some nice music and relax with a glass of wine before supper. Maria could tell that he had been upset and went along with his suggestion. The girls came in at that point and offered to make dinner, which Joe and Maria quickly accepted.

Later, when they went to bed, Maria quietly brought up the subject.

"You were acting funny when I got back from the store this afternoon. What happened?"

"I just got to thinking about what is happening and why is it happening to me. I got a little depressed, I guess."

He told her of some of the comments people had made, ostensibly while trying to cheer him up, and the fact that some of his friends appeared to be avoiding him.

"Yeah. I've heard of that from women who have breast cancer. Apparently people tend to personalize your disease to themselves, if you understand what I mean. But here I am doing it too. This is not about them or me. It's about the tribulations you are facing. Just know that I'm with you one hundred percent."

Joe knew Maria understood him. As he lay there, he could hear her gentle breathing and knew she was asleep. He thought about it longer, however, and prayed that things would work out, not so much for him, but for his family. They deserved it.

Websites Joe and Maria used to locate a proton beam treatment center

Note: for updated information on websites and other information in this book, please see www.RoadToNamiIsland.blogspot.com.

National Association for Proton Therapy (NAPT) - www.proton-therapy.org/

Blog on proton beam therapy option - http://affordableprotontherapy.blogspot.com/

Information from KMI International, an organization which facilitates patients going to the National Cancer Center in Seoul, Korea - http://www.internationalkmi.com/html/index.php

---

Following are the hospitals and other facilities with currently operating proton beam treatment centers (as of March 2012). For news and updates concerning the opening of new centers, see www.RoadToNamiIsland.blogspot.com.

James M. Slater, M.D. Proton Treatment and Research Center at Loma Linda University Medical Center, Loma Linda, California (USA) - www.protons.com/

The University of Florida Proton Therapy Institute, Shands Hospital, Jacksonville, Florida (USA) - www.floridaproton.org/

The University of Texas M.D. Anderson Cancer Center's Proton Center, Houston, Texas (USA) - www.mdanderson.org/about-us/index.html

ProCure Proton Therapy Center, located at the INTEGRIS Cancer Campus, Oklahoma City, Oklahoma (USA) - www.procure.com/OurLocations/Oklahoma.aspx

CDH Proton Center/ProCure Proton Therapy Center, near Naperville, Illinois (Suburban Chicago, USA) - www.procure.com/OurLocations/Illinois.aspx

The Roberts Proton Therapy Center at University of Pennsylvania Health System, Philadelphia, Pennsylvania (USA) - www.pennmedicine.org/perelman/

Hampton University Proton Therapy Institute, Hampton, Virginia (USA) - www.hamptonproton.org/

Francis H. Burr Proton Therapy Center, Massachusetts General Hospital, Boston, Massachusetts (USA) - www.massgeneral.org/radiationoncology/BurrProtonCenter.aspx

Indiana University Health Proton Therapy Center, Bloomington, Indiana (USA) - iuhealthprotontherapy.org/

Rinecker Proton Therapy Center, Munich, Germany - www.rptc.de/en/the-center.html

National Cancer Center/Proton Beam Therapy Center Korea, Seoul, South Korea - www.ncc.re.kr/english/proton/introduction.jsp

CHAPTER 5. KOREA

On Sunday evening it was Monday morning in Korea. The previous Friday Joe had talked to Mr. Curtis Poling, the representative in the United States for KMI, the company that handles marketing for the National Cancer Center. Mr. Poling had sent Joe an email indicating that based on his questionnaire he was a potential candidate for proton treatment. Joe had emailed his medical records, specifically including the biopsy results, and they had been forwarded to Korea by Mr. Poling.

Now that he had made a decision about getting treatment, Joe was anxious to get the project moving, but he realized that he was going to have to be somewhat patient. As he used to remind the girls as it was approaching some big event like Christmas "you can't push the clock."

Mr. Poling's email had given a rough estimate of the price for treatment and a brief explanation of what the package covered. It also explained that once he had been accepted for treatment and decided to proceed, he would be sent instructions on making a wire transfer of the funds and a date would be set. Joe decided that he should focus on logistics while he waited, so that there would be less to do once he was accepted.

On Monday morning, Joe called his insurance company to fill them in on the emerging details of the arrangements for his treatment. Since the insurance company would be reimbursing him for a portion of the cost, his plan was to borrow the portion that would be reimbursed and take the balance out of the money he had set aside for medical emergencies, along with a small amount from his retirement account. He had previously approached his bank to set this up. Accordingly, his next call was to his bank representative to provide him with the details of the estimated cost and payment arrangements. He told the banker that he would have final numbers when his case was accepted and he received the quote. The bank told him that the money would be ready to transfer electronically as soon as the arrangements were finalized.

Later in the day, Joe called Bill to fill him in on the evolving situation and to find out if there was any more news on Dennis. Bill was busy, but they agreed to meet for coffee at the end of the day.

When Joe reached the coffee shop, Bill had just arrived and had found them seats.

"So first, bring me up to date on Dennis," Joe started.

"I finally talked to him this weekend," Bill replied. "He has started the hormone therapy recommended by his urologist. He couldn't bring himself to try the chemotherapy because of the side effects. Barbara is still not very happy, but I think she is beginning to accept the situation and is willing to work with whatever Dennis decides."

Joe related what he had been doing to start the process of getting accepted for treatment by the National Cancer Center in Seoul. He told Bill what his tentative schedule might be for travel, although nothing was firm at this point.

As they were finishing their coffee, Bill suddenly jumped up. "Over here Mr. Kim," he called and motioned to a man coming in the door. "Can you join us?"

"Yes," the man answered. "Let me get a coffee."

When the man joined them, Bill made the introductions. "Mr. Kim, this is my good friend Joe. Joe this is Mr. Kim, who is a native of Korea. Perhaps he can tell you something about the country."

He explained to Mr. Kim that Joe had discovered that he had prostate cancer and had made the decision to seek proton beam treatment at the National Cancer Center in Seoul.

"I'm just starting the process of getting accepted for treatment there," explained Joe. "So far, I have had very little time to research Korea as a travel destination."

"Well, you are in for a treat," started Mr. Kim. "Of course, it is my homeland and I may be a little biased. I have had to travel a lot on business, and I have lived here in Argentina for the last several years. I enjoy it here, and I look forward to being assigned to live in the United States at some point, but I also look forward to getting home again someday. I think you will find the people in Korea to be very friendly and the country is aggressively modernizing, although there are still areas that are old and have not yet met the bulldozer. Most people speak at least some English, so you should not have too much trouble communicating. Do you know yet where you will be staying or where the treatment facility is located?"

Joe shook his head. "I have looked at a few websites, but I am still a little short on details. I have spoken to the international representative of the organization and he has shipped me a packet of information, but it has not arrived yet. I expect that I will be doing a lot of studying before I go, assuming that I get accepted."

The men chatted a little more. "Please call on me if you have any questions," said Mr. Kim, giving Joe his business card.

"I'm sure I'll have many questions. I appreciate the offer," said Joe.

They all said goodbye and went their separate ways.

On Wednesday Joe was at his office when the information packet arrived from Mr. Poling. The packet included information about the National Cancer Center and housing accommodations. It was accompanied by a packet of tourist information on things to see and do in Korea. Joe spent most of the afternoon studying the packet, and took it home to share with Maria. They spent the evening in their home office going over the materials and searching a number of websites related to the National Cancer Center, to the accommodation facilities, and to information about getting around and doing things in Korea.

On Saturday, Joe got an email from Mr. Poling indicating that the National Cancer Center had accepted Joe for treatment. With the email were instructions about making the wire transfer. The email also gave Joe the dates that were available. Joe showed the email to Maria, and then checked the calendar and sent an email back agreeing to the arrangement. He would have to wait until Monday to send the wire transfer, but he had plenty of other things to do in the meantime.

As he knew from earlier research and discussions, the price included all of the medical services related to the proton beam treatment, housing accommodations during his stay in Korea, and transportation between the airport and the residential facility. The price did not include transportation to Korea or incidental expenses and most meals while he was in Korea. Nor did it include regular daily transportation between the residence and the National Cancer Center for treatment.

Joe had already checked on flight schedules and airfares and was ready to make airline reservations. Joe had several choices of airlines and connections, with connections through North American cities or through European cities. Joe chose to travel through the United States, and selected a Saturday departure that took him on a non-stop overnight flight on Delta Air Lines from Buenos Aires to Atlanta, making a connection with another non-stop overnight flight operated jointly by Delta Airlines and Korean Air from Atlanta to Seoul.

The plan called for Joe to travel to Korea in early September for treatment lasting eight weeks. Ironically, as Joe was reviewing his schedule, he realized that September is Prostate Cancer Awareness Month. His stay would be nine weeks total to accommodate the week of orientation and pre-treatment tests, along with eight weeks of treatment. He would be returning in November, just before the American holiday of Thanksgiving. This schedule meant that he had almost four weeks between the day he got the formal notice that he was accepted and the day he would first appear at the National Cancer Center.

During these four weeks, Joe was active in making preparations and learning as much as he could about the experiences he was getting ready to have.

Joe did some Internet research on traveling to and living in Korea and made a few special arrangements. Among other things, he looked for information on how to get around in Korea and to find things he would need. One valuable resource was a web blog created by one of the many North Americans who live in Korea, primarily as English teachers. Another site he visited frequently was posted by the Korean Tourism Organization.

Another source was his daughter, Teresa, who helped him research Korea using the Internet. Teresa was still studying Asia and the Pacific Rim and had developed a particular interest in Korea. Teresa also read through the package of brochures and information Mr. Poling had mailed to Joe. From these sources, she had developed a list of places she thought Joe should visit in Korea and had asked that he send her lots of photographs.

Joe learned from his Internet research that the visa requirements had been changed, and that he would not need a visa for a stay less than ninety days. Joe calculated that he would not be in Korea that long and decided he would be okay since his passport was up to date.

He downloaded Skype and installed it on both his laptop and Maria's computers and while online purchased a microphone headset for each. He had read that this was the best way (in terms of quality and price) to communicate, as some cell phones are not compatible with the Korean cellular system. He also put a small amount of money into his Skype account so it could be used to call people who were not on Skype. The package by the National Cancer Center includes a cell phone with 300 minutes of time, but Joe decided to use that phone only in emergencies or when he was away from his computer. Joe also investigated online streaming TV options. The apartment provided by the National Cancer Center has cable and satellite TV but not all of the channels were ones he would normally select. In particular, he wanted to be prepared to watch American professional and college football - part of the United States he never left behind! He made sure he had the right cables so that he could stream shows directly from his computer into the TV set in the apartment.

Joe also knew from his research that the electrical system in Korea delivered the same voltage as was used in Argentina, but at a different frequency. This would not affect his laptop computer, which used a power adapter, but it might affect his electric shaver. He decided that the simple answer would be to just get a different shaver when he got there.

Joe made sure he had an adequate supply of medicines and personal items (particularly those where he had a strong brand preference) as these might be a little harder to find or prices on some items might be higher than he was used to paying. Joe did not want to have to spend his time in Korea searching for small items.

Joe was planning to travel in the fall, so he made sure he had a variety of clothing options. Korea is very cold in the winter and can be hot in the summer. There was little way of knowing what the coming fall would have in store, and Joe planned to be out and about a good bit, rather than being cooped up because of the weather. He decided to be prepared with some basic clothes, but be aware that he might need to purchase some additional clothes while he was there.

Finally, Joe studied the "won," the currency used in Korea and the rate of exchange. He realized that he would have to work to become familiar with the Korean currency, which was trading at about 285 to the Argentine peso (about 1180 to the U.S. dollar) in round numbers. This meant a taxi ride that might cost 40 pesos (a little more than 9.50 U.S. dollars) would cost about 11,400 won. To prepare for the trip, he arranged to get some cash in won, as well as a few American dollars to use while he was between planes in Atlanta. He had heard a general rule for international travelers was to avoid having to exchange currency at airports but to use banks.

Joe also took Mr. Kim up on his offer to provide information. He called the gentleman several times with questions he couldn't get answered on the Internet. Shortly before he left, he treated Bill and Mr. Kim to lunch to thank them both for their help.

When they had gathered at Bill and Joe's favorite restaurant near the tennis club, Joe again told Mr. Kim he appreciated his assistance.

"I have learned many things and have done a lot of reading and research since I first met you just a few weeks ago," Joe began. "Korea seems to be an amazing place, with a cross between centuries of culture and tradition, and the most modern facilities and lifestyle anywhere. I didn't know when I began my research that South Korea is the most 'wired' country in the world. More people are connected to the Internet than anywhere else. At the same time, the history of Korea is very turbulent. The people have been under a number of different rulers, including foreign rulers. It must be that the people have learned to be very resilient and that they have acquired the skill to adjust. I really look forward to visiting and seeing all the places there are in Korea."

Mr. Kim explained that he was originally from Busan, a major port city on the east coast of Korea.

"Busan is a major port for commercial and industrial goods, but it is also becoming a cruise port for many of the cruise lines that serve the western Pacific. Did you know that it also has the largest department store in the world?"

"I didn't know that," replied Joe. "I'll have to include a trip to Busan. How do I get there from Seoul, and how long will I need to plan?" Joe had a pad of paper ready to make notes. This was just like a business meeting.

They continued to discuss various areas and cities in Korea, outside of Seoul.

"I have a fair idea of the things I want to see in the immediate Seoul area, but I also want to use the few weekends I have to good advantage. It helps that South Korea is not huge, and you can almost literally get from one end to the other on the high-speed trains in only a few hours. I look forward to that."

Mr. Kim mentioned a few destinations Joe should try to see, including Pyeongchang, which had just been announced as the site of the 2018 Winter Olympic Games and would be a good weekend destination. He also suggested Nami Island which is closer to Seoul. He also mentioned Jinju, a city in southern Korea regarded as a center of traditional Korean culture and noted for tea ceremonies.

"Unfortunately, since you are confined mostly to weekends during your stay, you may have difficulty traveling to Jeju Island off the coast to the south. You can get there, but there is so much to see and do, you will not be able to do it justice. One of the ways you can get there is by ferry from Busan, which is a trip I recommend."

"Do you have any advice for me for Seoul, not necessarily tourist sites, but regular places?"

"You must experience the parks," said Mr. Kim. "I have been to many cities and I believe the parks are particularly nice in Korea. They are clean and safe and well maintained. They are high-tech, too. If you walk in the park in the evening, the lights will come on as you approach and go off again after you pass."

"Interesting," Bill and Joe exclaimed together. "I have to experience that," added Joe and made another note.

"Also," continued Mr. Kim, "if you enjoy tennis you will have to try out the many tennis clubs."

Joe made another note: "tennis racket."

"I'll have to mention that one to the girls," he said.

The topic switched to Joe's trip preparations. He told them about learning to mentally convert currency so he could figure quickly what something cost. He also described learning about the electrical system, and his study of subway maps, guidebooks, and online blogs.

When they were done, Joe promised Mr. Kim that he would contact him after he returned and let him know how his visit in Korea had gone.

Joe's travel itinerary called for him to depart Buenos Aires' Ministro Pistarini International Airport (referred to locally as Ezeiza International Airport) to Seoul (the new modern Inchon Airport). The first flight leg departed Buenos Aires in the evening, and Maria and the girls came to see him off. He arrived in the early morning in Atlanta and had a several hour layover until his flight left for Korea. The second leg of his journey departed in the early afternoon and involved crossing the International Date Line. Joe arrived in Korea on Monday in the late afternoon, two days after he left Buenos Aires, but by the time he arrived, it was only early Monday morning in Buenos Aires.

Joe understood that most patients arrive on Tuesday, just in time to have their medical consultation on Wednesday and their tests on Thursday. Joe planned to arrive late in the day on Monday, which made his schedule similar to the schedules of the other patients. He reasoned that the extra night would be just a little more time to help adjust to the extreme time change.

Even though passenger traffic appeared to be heavy, customs did not take very long. Joe was met at the airport by Wendy, his assigned concierge from the National Cancer Center, who connected with him as soon as he had cleared customs and then gave him a ride to the city. All during the ride he and Wendy kept up a light conversation. She pointed out several landmarks to Joe, while he observed the cityscape. He was impressed to see that Korea was certainly progressive, as he had been told by Mr. Kim. Many new buildings were being constructed and the city seemed to be characterized by higher density development, suggesting that public transportation would be good and he would be able to get around fairly easily even though he did not have a car. At the same time, Joe was almost dumbfounded by how large Seoul was. He had studied the maps, but thought to himself that nothing really prepared you for seeing it the first time.

As they traveled, Wendy explained that she had been assigned to Joe's case as soon as he had been accepted for treatment. She told Joe that she would handle all details of his trip and stay arrangements, including assistance with tour arrangements and general local information and assistance. The concierge also conducts orientations for the newcomers to make sure they can get around effectively. Joe knew he would be getting a lot of help from her during his stay. One of the things she explained was that since Korean names are typically difficult for westerners to remember and pronounce, many of the staff of the National Cancer Center had adopted westernized nicknames. This was not a derogation of the language or culture of Korea, but a pragmatic recognition of the need for clear communication.

The trip into Seoul took about an hour, and Joe arrived at his lodging by early evening.

The National Cancer Center had arranged an apartment that Joe would occupy for the duration of his treatment. Housing was included in the cost of the treatment, unlike programs in the United States.

Joe arrived and checked in. He was very impressed with his suite and took a good look around. The unit had two bedrooms, one that comfortably contained a double bed and had a walk-in closet. It also had two bathrooms, one with a tub and the other with a full-size shower. The rest of the apartment consisted of the kitchen (complete with dishes and cooking and serving utensils), a small eating area, and a living room with sofa, chairs, and a modern entertainment center. The apartment also had a washing machine. The master bedroom and living room opened through sliding-glass doors onto small balconies with a view of the bustling, modern city of Seoul.

Joe thanked Wendy and asked when she would do the orientation she had arranged. Wendy told him that normally they would do part of the orientation right after the patient arrives, but that due to the lateness of the hour, they would start the next day, and complete it on Friday after he was finished with his medical consultation and testing. She also told him that on Wednesday she would accompany him to the NCC to complete paperwork and to have his first consultation with the doctor. On Thursday, she would escort him to the NCC where he would spend most of the day undergoing tests. Joe and Wendy would finish the orientation on Friday, which would leave him the weekend to adjust to his new surroundings before treatments began. She told him the portion of the orientation for Tuesday would be a tour of the neighborhood to familiarize him with some of the nearby shops and services.

After she left, he unpacked his clothes and personal items and stowed his bags in the closet.

By then it was past 8 PM, which was 8 AM Monday, Buenos Aires time. Joe had slept and eaten on the plane, as he had no problem sleeping when he traveled, so he was not particularly tired or hungry. Also, his excitement about traveling to a new place and his expectation of getting his prostate cancer problem resolved kept him going. But Joe realized that he would need to adjust to Korean time, and the best way to do that would be to go to bed and wake up according to the local clocks.

Before he did, Joe set up his laptop and microphone/headset and placed a Skype call to Maria. He gave her a rundown of the trip and described the apartment, and told her he would call her again Tuesday night, which would be Tuesday morning for her. When he made his first call, the girls had already left for school, so he said he would call early enough on Tuesday to be able to speak to them. It was convenient that the time was just twelve hours different, so that it would be easy to make the calculation.

When he went to bed on his first night in Korea, Joe reflected on the journey he was taking; not only the journey to Korea, but the journey to overcome his prostate cancer. He noted that he was kind of at a midway point. It had been about two months since he found out that he might have a problem, and he was on schedule such that in about two months he would complete his treatments and would be on the path to resuming his normal life. Two months ago, he realized, he didn't even know what a PSA test was. And two months from now he would be returning to his wife and family.

He thought about the highs and lows he had been through emotionally. He had had several depressing moments, such as when he had been told he might have cancer, and then again when he learned he actually had it. He had spent a number of sleepless hours on some of the nights during that period. He thought also about the exhilarating feeling he had when he took charge of his situation, researched his options, and discovered proton beam therapy and the National Cancer Center. He also thought about how he felt when he received the email accepting him for treatment.

He reflected that it was like he was in an emotional valley, and that he had been climbing out of it and could see the hill in the distance, but knew that he could climb the hill and overcome his disease. As an engineer, he visualized this graphically. A deep "V" on paper represented the valley, and he was climbing up the right hand side of the "V" toward the top of the mountain. Soon he would reach the top and be able to see what lay beyond.

He also thought about the sights he had seen and the few people he had met during the short time he had been in Seoul. Wendy had escorted him from the airport to the DMC Ville apartment and had been especially helpful with practical information. He knew right away that he would be able to count on her for assistance and information to facilitate his stay in Korea. The staff at the DMC Ville had also been very helpful, letting him know what services and facilities were available. He knew that the help he would be getting from these people would contribute in a meaningful way to his treatment and eventual recovery.

He felt comfortable and in good hands.

Joe slept well and was awakened Tuesday morning by the alarm. He was anxious to get to the National Cancer Center to start the preparations for his treatment program. But that would come tomorrow; today would be devoted to becoming adjusted to the apartment and its facilities, as well as to learning all about the neighborhood. He also wanted to start mastering the challenge of finding his way around Seoul.

He showered and dressed, then went to the breakfast room the apartment supplied for use by its guests on weekdays. He would have to investigate and shop for groceries, as he planned to make many of his meals in his own kitchen.

After breakfast Joe took a quick tour of the apartment building. It had a fitness center providing a gymnasium, an aerobic exercise room, a private sauna, a twenty five-meter pool, a Jacuzzi, a driving range and putting greens, and two full sized squash courts. It also had an outdoor garden and a resident's lounge, as well as indoor and outdoor children's playgrounds.

Services included a 24-hour concierge, security and maintenance services, weekly housekeeping service, and weekday breakfast service, which Joe had just experienced.

For business people, it provided a multi-purpose conference room and secretarial and courier series.

Finally, Joe noted that it was conveniently located with respect to bus and subway lines and that shuttle service was also available to specific locations on a regular schedule. Among other things, he could catch the shuttle to the grocery store, which would make it easier to bring back his purchases. Even though the subway station was only about a mile away, he could also take a local bus to the subway station, where many other bus lines came together.

Today was scheduled for orientation, and he met Wendy in the apartment lobby. Since he had already taken a tour of the facilities in the building, they skipped that step and went straight to the tour of the neighborhood. Wendy showed Joe some of the facilities and services that were available in the area. A very short distance away he found that there was a convenience store, a chicken shop (Joe was especially interested in trying the Korean fried chicken, as he had read about it on the Internet), a Japanese grocery, and two coffee shops. In the nearby area there were also small restaurants and bars, as well as small Korean food markets.

Wendy explained to Joe that Koreans loved coffee shops and that there were many in Seoul. Several of the other patients who were staying at the DMC Ville met regularly in one such shop nearby to exchange information and to plan their exploring and leisure activities. This coffee shop was called TwoSomes, and sometimes referred to as "A TwoSome Place." She also pointed out that the DMC Ville was reserved for foreign visitors, including patients and business people, but that Koreans did not stay there. Joe asked where they stayed, and Wendy told him that most were from the Seoul area and simply commuted from home to the treatment facility. Those that were not from Seoul usually stayed with relatives or other lodgings that catered to Koreans.

Wendy then took Joe on the apartment shuttle to a much larger store about a mile away inside the World Cup Stadium and a short distance from the subway and bus stations. Wendy told him that this store, called HomePlus, was part of a chain and was useful because of the extensive line of goods it carried and because the DMC Ville shuttle made regular trips. Joe was pleasantly surprised by the extent of goods offered in this store. He found that they would not only sell you food, but you could purchase already cooked meals that you could take home. These were freshly made to order while you shopped. He later described it to Maria as a Super Wal-Mart on steroids.

One thing Joe noticed was how attentive the clerks and sales people were. He hardly had to pause to look at something when someone was there to help him. Most of the clerks in the store spoke at least some English.

Another thing Joe noticed was that many of the products had no English labels. He decided that as he learned about new products, he was going to need to be able to identify them by the color and appearance of the packaging when he wanted to get them again. Joe purchased some basics including cereal, coffee, canned juices, as well as a few snacks and interesting-looking Korean items. On the shuttle on the way back to the apartment, Wendy pointed out a few general merchandise shops, along with more restaurants. Joe was beginning to get a sense of where he would be able to get the things he would routinely need. He was impressed with the extent and variety of stores and services. He mentioned this to Wendy; she told him that he should be able to find almost anything he wanted in Seoul.

"You will come to realize how big a place this is," she said.

When they returned to the apartment, Wendy told him that there were four other proton patients currently staying at the DMC Ville. Two of them had been in Korea for about four weeks. The other two were starting at the same time as Joe. He might meet the other new patients either Wednesday or Thursday as they would likely be going to the proton center when he did. Wendy said that she would pick up Joe in the morning and escort him to the National Cancer Center for his orientation and his medical consultation appointments.

After she left, Joe decided to continue his tour of the neighborhood. Joe had a general map of the city, and the staff at the front desk gave him a flyer with a more detailed map of the area, listing various key facilities, including shops, convenience stores, coffee shops, restaurants, and entertainment venues. It was a pleasant late summer day, so Joe thought the walk would do him some good, helping to get over the confinement of the long airplane trip.

Joe's walk took him toward the nearest subway station (the Digital Media City station on line number 6 (the brown line), located about a mile east of the apartment. The station was referred to on the subway map as "Susaek" and was located between the World Cup Stadium and Jeungsan stations. He also noticed several bus stops along the way. He would have to get to know this information, particularly if he found himself lost and needed to get back. Along the way, Joe passed office buildings of a number of well-known international firms, as well as the Sangam Elementary and High School complex.

On his way back, Joe went by one of the small Korean markets and explored the merchandise. He noticed that in the smaller shops, fewer of the clerks spoke English, and concluded that these shops were less frequented by the foreigners who were staying at the apartment. When a particular clerk didn't speak enough English, however, there was usually someone else nearby who could step in and help. Joe also found the people he met to be very friendly. Joe decided his biggest challenge in communication would be finding out what certain items, particularly food items, were called and how they were supposed to be used. He decided that if he found something interesting at the store near the World Cup Stadium, he would ask that it be prepared and watch to see how it was done.

When Joe returned to his apartment, he put away his purchases and made a sandwich, then fiddled with the TV set and his laptop to set up some sort of streaming entertainment. This project went well enough, but he settled on CNN International and BBC, mainly to catch up with what was going on in the world. Joe was getting tired, and realized that the excitement of the trip and the anticipation of the upcoming cancer treatment were starting to take a toll and emphasized the need to transition to the local clock.

He called Maria at about seven so he could get a chance to speak with the girls. He brought them all up to speed on what he had done and learned that day. After the girls left for school, Joe let Maria know that he missed her and the girls, but that he was excited about the prospects for being rid of his cancer. He promised that he wouldn't call so early most of the time, but Maria said they would prefer that he call early on weekdays as the girls wanted to talk to him too.

Joe went to bed and had another good night's sleep, awakening to the alarm at seven. He decided to follow his daily sleep-wake schedule, as he had already learned that his regular appointments would be scheduled for the same time: ten o'clock each morning. Until he was adjusted and had experienced the treatment and confirmed that there were no side effects, Joe had decided not to do any late partying. He got up, showered, dressed, and went downstairs for breakfast.

Wednesday's main order of business was to meet with his doctor to discuss his treatment. Wendy met him in the apartment lobby and escorted him to the NCC. Joe had also been instructed to bring the biopsy slides with him. He turned these over to the doctor when they met the consultation.

"We have carefully reviewed the medical information you previously submitted," said the doctor. "Tomorrow you will take a series of tests so that we can design your treatment program. Your treatments will begin next Monday morning."

The doctor went on to explain the treatment procedure. "Each day you will come into the Center and will be prepared for the treatment session. You will need to drink about a pint of water a half hour before your treatment. This fills your bladder and holds your prostate gland in a stable position which steadies it and guarantees a more accurate delivery of the proton dose. Then you will change into a hospital gown and at the time of the treatment, you will be taken into the gantry room. The gantry is a giant rotating device that can assume almost any position to aim the proton beam at the cancer target. Both you and the gantry will be positioned for the treatment dose using the Digital Image Positioning System (DIPS). The treatment itself will take about three minutes, after which you will go back into the dressing room where you will change back into your street clothes and will be released for the day. Once a week you will meet with me and we will review the status of your treatments and I will be able to answer any questions you might have."

Joe had a question. "What exactly will I feel, and what side effects will there be?"

The doctor replied: "You will not feel anything during the treatment itself. You may be a little tired and you may have a mild discomfort when you urinate. You may have increased urgency and frequency when you urinate, but these will all go away within a few weeks after treatment. Those people who drive to the Center for treatment find that they can easily drive back and forth for their treatment sessions. Long-term side effects are very rare and you should be able to enjoy a normal life after the treatments have been completed."

"What about incontinence and erectile dysfunction?" Joe asked. He believed that he already knew the answer, but he wanted to hear it again.

"That is one of the primary advantages of proton beam therapy," replied the doctor. "Unlike surgery and x-ray, or photon radiation, the proton beam does very little disturbance to the surrounding tissues and does not injure them. We do not experience the 'slip of the knife' nor do we have secondary cancers or other conditions caused by photon radiation that will require long-term treatment and care. Once the treatment has been completed and the cancer has been removed, you should not have any additional ill effects."

"Will I need to return to the Center in Korea after my treatment is complete?" Joe asked.

"No. Of course we will continue to monitor your progress by reviewing blood test information that will be collected at your own doctor's office at home," answered the doctor.

As he had planned to do each evening, Joe called Maria and the girls. He had many new things to tell them about the NCC and the things the doctor said, but he realized that he missed their family tradition of sharing experiences. He decided to make sure they got to tell first the next day when he called.

Joe turned in early. He noticed that he was adjusting to the time change, and would probably be acclimated by the weekend.

Joe's formal activities for Thursday at the National Cancer Center included a series of tests and required most of the day. While he would not need to return until the following Monday to begin his therapy, the next couple of days would be spent by the technicians and doctors at the National Cancer Center in refining his treatment plan and making the customized diffuser to be used in shaping the beam for his own therapy.

Waiting in the lobby for Wendy and the driver to take him to the NCC, Joe met two new patients who were scheduled to start treatments at the same time as he was. Joe later found out that these men were referred to as being in his "class," which meant that their treatment schedule coincided with his.

One gentleman introduced himself as Mr. Morgan, a citizen of South Africa. The other was Mr. Bailey, an Englishman living in Singapore.

Mr. Bailey indicated he had arrived at the DMC Ville at the end of the previous week, and had had an opportunity to meet some other patients. "There is a Mr. Bentley from the United States, and a Mr. Charles from France. They have each been here about four weeks and consider themselves to be old hands, but they are not stuffy about it," he explained. "I suspect we will run into them at TwoSomes. The proton patients seem to congregate there to socialize, although socializing generally involves discussion of PSA levels, Gleason scores, and staging."

They only had a brief time to talk before they arrived at the National Cancer Center, but they agreed to meet later to exchange information.

At the National Cancer Center Wendy described the activities that would take place that day and took him on a very brief tour of the Center.

The schedule for this day involved a battery of tests, including a CT scan and an MRI "primarily for the purpose of designing the proton treatment protocol," explained the technician. "We will also do a CT scan prior to each treatment. The scan will be used to establish and confirm the aiming coordinates and the dosage levels for the treatment."

"Based on the information we get from these scans and from the tests," he continued, "we will also make tattoo marks on your body to help fix the aiming points. We will create an immobilization device to be used to keep your body still so that the aiming will be most effective."

Joe observed that the "tattoo" consisted of making marks with a permanent laundry marker. He was glad that it wasn't a real tattoo, but was ready to ask if they could add the word "Maria."

Joe was finished about four in the afternoon. Wendy escorted him to the car and driver, which took him back to the apartment.

Friday was scheduled for more orientation. Since much of the introduction to local shops and services had been covered on Tuesday, Friday was focused on how to use the subway and bus systems. Joe had already done extensive research on this and was a good student, so the lesson went quickly.

When they concluded the bus and subway orientation, Wendy gave him a set of cards with English/Korean translations of useful words and phrases, primarily to be used in giving directions or getting assistance. An example was a card that gave the name and address of the DMC Ville, so that he would be able to communicate with a non-English speaking taxi driver to tell him he wanted to go to the DMC Ville. Another example was a card that he could use to ask a stranger how to get to the nearest subway station. The cards were strung on a cord to keep them together. Joe thought to himself that these might be referred to as directions-on-a-rope.

Joe felt he was generally acclimated to the immediate environs of the DMC Ville and the subway system. He felt he was ready to launch his Korea plan. Before he made the trip, Joe had spent some time studying websites and reading books from the library, as well as the materials Mr. Poling had mailed to him. From this information, and with Teresa's help, Joe had made a plan for his weekends with the intention of seeing and experiencing as much as he could during the duration of his stay. He had even reviewed his plan with Mr. Kim to determine if it was too ambitious. Mr. Kim thought it was reasonable as far as the logistics of it went but that Joe might become worn out by the level of activity he was planning for himself.

His plan was to use his first weekend to become as familiar as he could with the full extent of Seoul and how to get around efficiently. He already knew that Seoul was a big place, with many forms of transportation, and that if you didn't familiarize yourself with the basic system and make appropriate preparations, you could get lost. Wendy's basic training lessons had familiarized him with the basics of the subway and bus systems.

He had already figured out that it would be better to stay with the subway system until he became more comfortable with the bus system. The subway system is better marked and has signs in Korean and English (as well as Chinese and Japanese in some cases), while the bus system, though extensive, is largely signed in Korean. Furthermore, there were a number of different bus systems, using different colored busses. The subway system follows fixed routes easily found on maps, while the bus system goes everywhere.

With some help from Wendy, Joe had studied the bus system, however, and learned that busses come in four colors to distinguish the different functional systems (red, yellow, blue and green). He worked at learning the distinctions.

Red buses go to the outskirts of the city, operating along many local routes. Yellow buses operate through the heart of the city. Blue buses operate on major arterial roads. Green buses operate on branch lines and their major role is to carry passengers to junctions. He also learned that each bus system had a system for numbering busses that indicated the area where the route began and ended.

Joe spent the rest of Friday seeking to expand his horizons by riding the subway as far as he could in several directions to see where it would take him and to become familiar with the way to get to some of the destinations that he would later be visiting. Also, since about 30 percent of the system involved above-ground lines, he figured that it would be a good way to get a feel for the arrangement of the larger city and to see some sights. Joe had realized that he would be making heavy use of the public transportation systems. Wendy had showed him how to buy a T- money card. The T-money card can be purchased directly from a street vendor, subway stations, and T-money member stores. The T-money card can be reloaded and is used not only for public transportation, but also for taxis, convenience store and vending machine purchases, and Internet cafés. Wendy also helped Joe purchase a prepaid ticket that could be used to pay fares on the Seoul subway system. The ticket cost 39,600 won (about $33.50 US) and can be used for up to 60 rides within 30 days of its purchase.

Joe found that the maps and color-coding made navigating the subway system much easier than he had anticipated. He was beginning to notice that many advertisements for destinations (such as stores or tourist sites) gave the color and/or number of the line that served the location, the name of the station, and even the exit number to use from the station. This was based on a system where each station has multiple exits that are all numbered to facilitate navigating from the station to the correct location on the street. Joe had had the experience of riding a subway in American cities, like Atlanta and Washington DC, and arriving at the correct destination station, only to get completely lost by going out the wrong exit.

Joe's call home on Friday evening was a welcome event on both ends of the line. Everyone in the whole family was excited by the fact that he would begin treatment on Monday. Each evening, he had described every step in detail and Maria was anxious to hear it all. He even described the device they inserted in his rectum to stabilize his prostate. He told her that since it was custom made, it was his to keep. She giggled. Each night, he also described some new place he had been or some new thing that he had done.

"There is something of a culture shock coming here," he explained to Maria. "I expected to run into centuries-old costumes and traditions. But what I didn't expect to see is all the technological innovation, which is another form of culture shock. I suppose some of this is the result of how much of the city has been built or rebuilt in such a short time. And little things are so different. For example, in the modern apartments and hotels you don't have light switches on the walls like we are used to. When you come in, you slide your plastic room key card into a slot and the lights come on throughout the apartment. When you leave, you remove the card and the lights all go off. Also, the air-conditioning is in wall units, but the heat is all in the floor slab. You have to figure out how to control it. One of the other patients said he didn't figure it out right away and wound up barely being able to walk around in his apartment because the floor was so hot. Oh, and I figured out how to run the washer, but it took me awhile to figure out how to make it dry my clothes."

Joe spent a good part of his first Saturday riding the trains and getting used to the extent of the system. As an engineer, he also was interested in some of the construction features of the system and studied how the problems of designing such an extensive system in three dimensions were handled.

He came out of the system at several points, exploring areas near monuments and other points of interest that he would be visiting later. These preliminary visits included the National Museum, the War Memorial of

Korea, and the Dongdaemun Market. He wanted to see these sights and to learn more about the history and culture of Korea (which turned out to be much more complex than he would have thought only a couple of months ago). But his ulterior motive was to practice identifying a destination he wanted to visit and then see how efficient he could be in getting there.

At the end of his first Saturday excursion, Joe went back to the apartment, stopping to get some milk and a few other things. Again, he had stretched his day as long as he could and was tired, but with a good feeling. He ate and called his wife and daughters, and was able to speak to the girls. He was starting to wish that he could be with them, but he knew what he had to do first.

Sunday morning, Joe woke up, showered, and decided to find a coffee shop or restaurant. First he logged onto his laptop, went to ESPN web site, and found the college football scores from Saturday afternoon (the late games weren't finished yet).

Joe went to A TwoSome Place and bought an English-language newspaper. Although most of the local news dealt with topics about which he knew little, it was nice to sit at a table, drink coffee and peruse the paper.

As he sat, Mr. Morgan and Mr. Bailey came by and he asked them to join him. Each man then gave a short explanation of his situation. Joe discovered that it was true - when men with prostate cancer get together, they often discuss their diseases, talking in terms of PSA levels, Gleason scores, and staging. Joe asked the others how they had discovered proton beam therapy and elected to go to Korea.

Mr. Bailey, the Englishman, went first. "When I was first diagnosed, the doctors in the national health system advised me to pursue the 'watchful waiting' strategy. I had a brother who did that and died, and I wasn't about to accept that fate. So I went online and found blogs and websites that gave me the information I needed. Long and short of it, this was the place where I could get treated the quickest for the cheapest, so I opted for it."

Mr. Morgan then explained that he had surgery on the advice of his doctor, but it hadn't removed all his cancer. At that point he did additional research on his own and discovered that proton can be used for salvage treatment in some cases, so he decided to go with proton.

After Joe told his story, they switched briefly to the topic of what each did for a living. Mr. Morgan was retired and a lover of the outdoors, particularly fishing. Mr. Bailey was a computer systems engineer. He explained that his company had agreed to assist with the cost of his treatment if he would continue to work on a part-time basis while he was in Korea.

"I find I am able to work about twenty to thirty hours a week on my laptop, connected to my computers at the office through the Internet. When I need to participate in a meeting, I use Skype, which works very well for both large and small groups."

Joe suddenly realized that this was a new dimension to his possibilities. He had not expected to be able to work much while he was away from his office. While this was not significant because his business had been slow anyway, if it turned out that there was any need to conduct a meeting, he could have the others go on Skype and include him. He resolved to email his assistant and advise her of this approach.

"What are you doing today?" Mr. Bailey asked Joe.

"I think I'll continue exploring. I have committed to myself that I will understand this city as soon as I can so that I can really take advantage of what it has to offer."

"We are planning to attend the football game at the World Cup Stadium. Would you care to come with us? We understand that the local team is very competitive and the opponent is one of their biggest rivals."

"No thanks," replied Joe. "I will check out attending a future game, but I have my day pretty well planned. Also I want to get back fairly early. I'm tired and at the same time excited about tomorrow."

"We understand," said Mr. Morgan.

For his trip of the day on Sunday, Joe took the subway to visit the COEX Mall, located near the Korean World Trade Center on the south side of the Hangang River. The mall was not the largest one he had ever seen, but it had an interesting diversity of facilities, including a number of American stores and restaurants. Joe decided he would try to stick with Korean choices if he could help it. After all, when in Rome…

Following his newly developing routine, Joe called his wife and daughters on Skype and related his experiences. An idea was forming in his mind that he might want to take a trip to Korea in the future and bring the family. He was beginning to really enjoy the place.

Websites Joe used in getting information on visiting Korea for medical treatment

Note: for updated information on websites and other information in this book, please see www.RoadToNamiIsland.blogspot.com.

Korea Tourism Organization (KTO) - This is the website for the official tourist organization of the Korean government, and has many useful links, including tour packages, visa and customs information, currency exchange information, etc. - http://asiaenglish.visitkorea.or.kr/ena/index.kto

Blog created to assist American and Canadian teachers who travel to Korea as teachers of English - http://thedailykimchi.blogspot.com/

Information from KMI International, an organization which facilitates patients going to the National Cancer Center in Seoul, Korea - http://www.internationalkmi.com/html/index.php

Information from KMI International on services and pricing - http://www.internationalkmi.com/html/we_price.php

Website of the National Cancer Center in Seoul, Korea - www.ncc.re.kr/english/proton/introduction.jsp

Wikipedia articles on Korea including articles on money exchange, travel, electric service, etc.

CHAPTER 6. TREATMENT IN KOREA

After a sunny and warm weekend, Monday came in with a drizzle and a noticeable chill. You could tell that fall and winter were on the way. Joe woke and showered. While excited about the prospect of dealing with his cancer, he was also a little nervous so he skipped the breakfast provided by management and just had some juice instead. He had been advised that eating before the treatment wasn't a good idea as it might cause gas. He was more than willing to put off his first meal of the day until later.

Joe took the car to the NCC hospital, arriving by nine. He was the only passenger, and he reasoned that both Mr. Morgan and Mr. Bailey had different treatment times. At the NCC he met Wendy who escorted him to the first stop in the patient preparation area. There she turned him over to the patient preparation staff. She told him she would meet him after his treatment and make sure he got back to the apartment properly.

The treatment process was in three parts: the patient was prepared for the treatment, the treatment was carried out, and the patient was removed from the preparation devices and returned to normal condition so that he could leave.

His first step was to drink his pint of water. It was desirable that he drink the water about thirty minutes before his treatment so that it would be in his bladder at the correct time.

The rest of the preparation consisted of Joe removing his clothes and donning a hospital gown. When he went into the gantry room, he lay down on the support, and technicians immobilized him with blocks and with a custom shaped device inserted into his rectum. They also positioned the beam with a laser pointed aimed as his magic marker tattoos and used a CT scan to further position the beam. During the treatment, Joe's body would have to be totally immobilized so that the proton beam could accurately target his tumor.

When everything was ready, the technicians went to the computer control room. Joe was completely alone, and for a moment had visions of Dr. Frankenstein's laboratory. He could almost hear Boris Karloff's chuckle.

The treatment process itself only took a few minutes, after which the technicians returned and removed the blocks and immobilization devices, and he was able to put back on his street clothes. The technicians then went to work setting up for the next patient.

Total time for the treatment, including all the preparation and post-treatment activity, was about an hour and fifteen minutes. Joe was driven back to the apartment, then went to a small restaurant near the DMC Ville to pick up a carry-out lunch. He realized that he was hungry since he had not eaten breakfast, but to be safe in case there were any side effects of the treatment, he ate a small meal and put the leftovers in his refrigerator for later.

After lunch Joe watched a little TV. He suddenly realized that it was early morning Monday in the Western Hemisphere, so he went online and checked the pro football scores from Sunday's games and the final results of the weekend golf tournaments. He marveled that he had gone a whole week and had forgotten about sports news.

Later in the afternoon Joe went out and took a walk around the neighborhood, picking up some interesting Korean food for supper and purchasing a couple of paperback mysteries and a tourist guide book.

That evening when he called Maria, and after the girls had left for school, he described in detail the treatment process. He included the part about Dr. Frankenstein's lab.

"I didn't feel a thing. Really, for all I know they just shined a flashlight on me. The only problem I had was that they slather on a lot of petroleum jelly or something like that in order to put this device in, and it gets all over my legs, so I really need to come straight back to the apartment and take a shower. But if that's all the price I have to pay, I am more than happy with the process."

Just like the first day on a new job is always the longest, and the first week is the longest, Joe's first week of treatment seemed to take forever. When he was working with the doctors on his treatment plan, Joe wished that he could take a treatment every day, or even twice a day, so that the total process would go faster. They explained to him, however, that the down time (weekends and from midnight to five every morning) was used by technicians to adjust and calibrate the machinery, which was very sensitive. Even though he did not feel anything, they told him, his body needed rest between sessions of therapy. Once in a while he might miss a day due to equipment problems, but this should not affect the overall treatment schedule.

By the end of the first week of treatment Joe had settled into a routine. He got up and showered, had some juice, checked online for the news from Argentina and sports results from the United States, used the provided car and driver to get to the NCC hospital, and underwent treatment. Periodically before he left the NCC, he would confer with the doctors and take additional tests so the doctor could monitor progress. Then he would take the car back to the apartment, shower, and have lunch. Joe had every afternoon to himself and worked from his plan to see and experience as much of Seoul as he could. He read and checked tourist guides and maps and, depending on the weather, he went out three or four afternoons a week. So far he had not succumbed to the temptation to go out and party, even though he had plenty of free time and he felt great, with no side effects from the treatments.

When he went out in the afternoon, he usually planned to return no later than seven so he could call home before the girls left for school. But this only happened when he went some distance; most of his trips got him back to the apartment by five or six, even though this required him to travel in the evening rush hour.

On weekends the call would be in the morning or evening, or both, depending on his and their schedules. In the evening after the call, Joe would watch a little TV or read. One evening, he had tired of both those pursuits, and suddenly hit on another option; there were websites that he could use to get streaming audio from radio stations around the world. He found his favorite easy-listening station in Buenos Aires and listened to it, staying up later than he should have. He found this was always the best strategy when he felt a little homesick.

Among other places in the Seoul area Joe visited during the next several weeks were Gyeongbokgung Palace, Deoksugung Palace, the Hangang River, Gwanghwamun Plaza, and the Moonlight Rainbow Fountain (Banbo Bridge). He also visited districts where shopping areas were located, including Itaewon.

Several destinations he found were so interesting that he had to go more than once in order to investigate them thoroughly. One of these was the North Seoul Tower, which on clear days allowed an exceptional view of Seoul and its surroundings. Joe found that after he visited a new area (and sometimes before) a trip to the Tower helped him gain a better perspective on where the destination was and how it related to other parts of Seoul.

He also took a number of guided tours, again to help him become familiar with places he would like to visit and to see things he might otherwise miss.

Some of these sights were better experienced in the evening, so Joe sometimes stayed in for the afternoon before venturing out. On these occasions, he would email Maria and let her know that he would be calling late, but he always called.

On weekends, Joe had two days to himself and he sometimes used those occasions to make longer trips out of town, usually leaving early on Saturday morning and returning late Saturday night or even staying at his destination overnight. When he knew he was going to be out of town Joe made sure Wendy and the front desk knew he would be gone, where he was planning to go, and when he would be back. Wendy gave him a lot of advice on locations to visit, methods of getting to his destination, and hints on what to look for and sights to visit.

Sometimes Joe would plan his trip himself, relying on his growing understanding of the country's extensive transportation system along with the guide books he had acquired and studied. Sometimes he would base his itinerary on one suggested by one of the many guide books he had studied. On other occasions, he would take a commercial tour, which usually provided the transportation, the itinerary, and the guide.

On the second weekend (the weekend after his first week of treatment), Joe took advantage of a package one-day tour to Panmunjom. A few days before he took the Panmunjom tour, Joe ran into Mr. Morgan and Mr. Bailey in the lobby after he returned from treatment.

"What have you guys been up to?" asked Joe. "I see you from time to time, but mostly when you're hurrying out and I'm hurrying in. Did you get your treatments started on schedule?"

"We're on our way there now," answered Mr. Bailey, the Englishman. "That's why we see you coming when we are going. We have our appointments scheduled in the afternoons."

"I just enjoy sleeping in," added Mr. Morgan, the South African. "Bailey here uses the time to work."

"I am able to do my work on the computer in the mornings, when the people in my office in Singapore are working," said Mr. Bailey. "That way I can communicate with them on a convenient schedule. How about you, Joe, what are you up to?"

Joe explained that he had been using his afternoons to explore Seoul and that he was planning to start expanding his travels to include other locations in Korea.

"I'm planning to go to the Demilitarized Zone this weekend. It will just be a day trip. I'm going on one of the many escorted tours since I want to be sure not to miss anything. And to make sure I don't wind up in the wrong country," he added with a chuckle.

They all smiled.

"We'd like to find out more about that," said Mr. Bailey, "but we have to get going. We have found out that many of the patients meet at the coffee shop across the street in the late afternoon. Can you join us there at about 7 this evening and tell us more about the trip?"

"I sure can," replied Joe.

When they had left, Joe realized that this was why he hadn't seen them around that much. They went to the proton center at the NCC in the afternoons after he had returned, then spent time at the coffee shop when he was returning from his afternoon excursions and heading to his apartment. He realized that it would be valuable to sit in on the coffee shop discussions as he might learn not only about the treatments but would be able to find out more about what to see and do in Korea. He emailed Maria to let her now his call would be a little late on this day and he would explain why when they talked.

Joe ate a light supper, planning to have coffee and perhaps dessert at the coffee shop. When the time came to go, he gathered up the brochures he had on the Demilitarized Zone tours and took them to the coffee shop.

Mr. Morgan and Mr. Bailey were already there and welcomed Joe when he arrived. They had been discussing the idea of getting out on the coming weekend, since neither one had done as much sight-seeing as had Joe.

Joe showed them the brochures, which explained the various sites that were included in the tour. They agreed that they wanted to go too. Mr. Morgan said he would call the tour agency in the morning and add his and Mr. Bailey's names to the Saturday tour.

The Demilitarized Zone tour took them to an observatory, one of North Korea's infiltration tunnels, a military base, and right into Panmunjom, the Joint Security Area in the middle of the DMZ. This was where negotiations between the two sides are held. Joe made sure he got lots of pictures. He realized that he wasn't sure if he would get another chance to go to some of these places and wanted to document his travel very well and send lots of pictures to Teresa.

They found out some interesting things. For one, even though the area surrounding the Demilitarized Zone (DMZ) includes some of the most military-intensive areas in the world, and the border between North and South Korea is one of the most heavily guarded, it is actually very safe. Another thing Joe learned was that because there is almost no human activity within the DMZ itself; it has become a wildlife preserve with significant bio-diversity.

The tour returned late in the evening to Seoul, so Joe called his wife on Sunday morning, when it was Saturday evening in Buenos Aries. Afterwards Joe caught part of a late college football game on ESPN, and then went to the coffee shop to read the paper and drink coffee.

At the coffee shop, Joe ran into Mr. Morgan and Mr. Bailey.

"Well good morning, Joe," said Mr. Bailey. "Guess what we're going to do today. We have decided to attend another football contest ('soccer' to you Americans) at the World Cup Stadium. Would you care to join us?"

Joe readily agreed.

The day was clear and cool, beautiful fall weather. The stadium was about a mile from the apartments so they decided to walk, or more correctly, stroll to it. They arrived in plenty of time and took their seats. It was obvious that the crowd was really energized for the game that was against a long-time rival team. Having lived for many years in South America, Joe was very familiar with football (although he still called it "soccer.") His daughters had played the game as they were growing up and he had been to professional games on more than one occasion with the contractors he worked for. While still mainly a fan of American football, Joe had to admit that there was a certain simplicity and efficiency to soccer. The game was close all the way and the home team scored in the last three minutes and held off a couple of severe challenges by the opponents to eke out the win. The crowd was thrilled and Joe was very glad he had agreed to come.

Joe realized that the thing most Americans don't get when it comes to soccer is that there is action all over the field away from the ball, and that the plays being set up by the teams and the strategies they reflected were just as interesting, if not more so, than the scoring plays themselves. In this respect, Joe thought, soccer was a lot like American baseball, where the nuances of what was going on around the playing field was often as interesting as the duel between the pitcher and the batter. While he was growing up, Joe attended many baseball games with his father, who had played minor league baseball in his youth. From time to time, Joe's father would say things like "watch the man on second. The third base coach is getting ready to have him steal third."

On the way back to the apartments, Mr. Morgan and Mr. Bailey introduced Joe to a small bar nearby. Joe had walked past this establishment many times on his walks and errands but had not gone in. The bar was occupied by its share of happy football fans, reveling in the victory. They found seats in a corner and ordered three bottles of soju. Mr. Morgan explained that soju is a favorite of both Koreans and non-Koreans. It is made primarily of rice and has a taste similar to that of vodka, although is a little sweeter. He also explained that there are certain customs when drinking soju, although he clarified that his information was largely from Wikipedia and that these customs actually applied to any beverage.

He explained that, among other things, you should not fill your own glass but wait for someone else to fill it. It is considered a good thing to fill someone else's empty glass, but they won't fill it unless it is actually empty. If your glass is to be filled by a superior, you should hand it to him using two hands, and if you are filling the glass of an elder you should hold the bottle with two hands. If an older person hands you an empty glass, it is an indication that he or she wants to fill the glass for you and you are to drink it. If you empty the glass, you return it to the person who gave it to you, but don't return it too early or take too long, both of which are impolite.

"Whew," said Joe. "That's a lot to remember."

Mr. Morgan continued. "Ah, there's more, but I won't go into it. Just be aware that there are many conventions in Asian countries. Make sure you look it up before you need to go to a social occasion."

"I'll do that," replied Joe.

They ordered some Korean fried chicken and one more round of soju, after which Joe excused himself and went back to the apartments. Joe called Maria and turned in. It had been a long day and tomorrow was the beginning of his second week of treatment.

Joe's second week of treatment was generally a copy of the first. He was getting used to his schedule and he still did not experience any side effects. He also continued his practice of visiting places throughout the immediate Seoul area, saving the longer trips for the weekends. To his schedule he added the routine of going several afternoons or early evenings each week to A TwoSome Place coffee shop. He discovered that the prostate cancer patients frequently turned from their various conversation topics to the topic of their cancers and their treatments.

On the second weekend, Joe decided to lie low, since the National Foundation Day holiday was coming up and he wasn't sure how this might impact travel. Instead, he stayed in Seoul, making another trip on Saturday to the National Museum of Korea. Joe had been here on his first weekend, but the object of that trip was to learn to get around Seoul. At the time he realized that he would be back when he had more time to explore.

Joe found that this is a place where people can explore the essence of Korean arts and culture. The museum combines Korean history, life, and arts. Exhibits range from hand axes of the Paleolithic period, to celadons (ceramics) of the Goryeo dynasty, to paintings of the Joseon dynasty, to modern photography. They provide docents to give tours in six different languages and offer a free one-hour guided tour in English twice a day.

Joe also found out that the National Museum of Korea was the ninth most-visited museum in the world in 2010, according to Art Newspaper. Joe concluded that it was impossible to take in the National Museum in one trip, and over the two months of his stay went at least five times.

"I actually lost count," he told Maria a few weeks later during one of their daily calls.

On Sunday of that weekend Joe traveled to the Insa-dong section. This is a center of art and culture, with interesting architectural and historic sites, and is a favorite destination of tourists. The area is also regarded as a highpoint of tradition and Korean culture. Joe made sure he took plenty of pictures of the buildings and street activities and sent them to Teresa when he got back to his apartment.

National Foundation Day, or Gaecheonjeol, celebrates the foundation of Gojoseon, the first state of the Korean nation. The modern Korean nation was established in 1949 following World War II. National Foundation Day, observed on October 3, celebrates the creation of Gojoseon in 2333 BC and is treated as the national birthday of Korea. Interestingly, Joe found out that the original celebration was based on the lunar calendar, but was changed to October 3 of the Gregorian calendar. National Foundation Day is a National Flag Raising Day, a National Celebration Day, and a Public Day Off, meaning that the NCC would not be operating that day.

On the third weekend, Joe had decided to take one of the bullet trains. Actually, the term bullet train is not used in Korea. The system is called the KTX, which stands for Korea Train Express. The technology of the early models is based on the French TGV trains. Based on his conversations with Mr. Kim, Joe chose to try out the service on the Seoul to Busan route, the original and longest one. Busan is on the southeast coast, a distance of just over 255 miles from Seoul, and is a major seaport. The trip takes just over 2 hours, including stops. This particular route serves a high-population corridor, representing about three-quarters of Korea's population.

Joe planned to go on Saturday, tour the city, and return early Sunday afternoon. Among other things, he would visit the world's largest department store, the Shinsegae Centum City, as well as other sites. Busan was the site of several international sporting events, including some of the games in the World Cup soccer tournament. Busan was also a major seaport and was becoming an active port of call for cruise ships.

Wendy helped him get tickets, make hotel reservations, and plan his tour of Busan.

This was Joe's first overnight trip out of Seoul. He was excited when he got back to the DMC Ville on Sunday afternoon and could hardly wait to make his call to Maria and the girls and tell them all about it. Prior to calling, he transferred all his photographs to his laptop and emailed them to Teresa. Later he described them all to her when he made the call.

On Tuesday evening during his fourth week of treatment, Joe attended the graduation party for Mr. Charles and Mr. Bentley, the two patients who had been in the program a few weeks before Joe arrived. The two had completed their treatment successfully and were getting ready to leave Korea for home. Joe was a little surprised when he noticed how somber the two men were, especially when they said their farewells to the NCC staff. Then he realized that he too was becoming fond of the staff and all the skill and care they were giving to him and his case. He would probably have some of the same feelings when it came time for him to leave.

Joe's original plan called for him to travel on the fourth weekend to Pyeongchang to see the locations where the 2018 Winter Olympics are to be held. The announcement that Pyeongchang had been selected had been made just before Joe left for Korea. He decided to postpone this trip until later in his visit, however. For one thing, Pyeongchang is a winter sports center and it wasn't winter yet. He expected that if he delayed, there might be more of an opportunity to see snow in the higher elevations.

Instead, Joe took local transportation to Imjingak, sometimes referred to as the Shrine to the Displaced. Imjingak is close enough to Seoul to be served by hourly commuter trains. Located only a few miles from the Military Demarcation Line, Imjingak is a central location for tourism related to the Korean Conflict. This is the closest most people can get to the DMZ without special permission. Joe took one of the tours, which were conducted in Korean. Having not mastered the language, Joe latched onto a group of American teachers who were working in Korea teaching English. They translated for him and he got along fine. He realized, however, that he would need to be a little more careful in selecting some of the places he went to overcome his lack of proficiency with the language. While the directions-on-a-rope helped considerably in many situations, they weren't sophisticated enough to accommodate complex conversations.

Joe checked out the exhibits and watched as North Koreans on the north side of the Imjigang River performed ancestral rites on behalf of their family members living in the South. He also purchased some North Korean food and gifts in the gift shop at the park.

On Wednesday evening during the week, Joe made his regular evening call to Maria. He spoke briefly with the girls just before they left for school, wishing them a good day. When they had gone, Maria changed the subject.

"Bill called last night and said there was a problem with Dennis. They've taken him to the hospital. He's leaving tonight to go up there. He's anxious to talk to you if he can. He went in to the office early this morning to get some paperwork done and he said to have you call him directly there." She gave Joe the direct number to Bill's office.

"Okay," said Joe. "I've kind of been expecting something like this, but I had hoped it wouldn't happen this soon. I'll call him as soon as we finish."

They exchanged goodbyes and hung up.

Joe then placed a call to Bill, who answered almost immediately.

"Joe, thanks for calling. Maria told me about your calling schedule and I know how prompt you are. I'll make it brief. Barbara called me last evening. Dennis wasn't well, so they took him to the hospital late in the afternoon yesterday. It turns out that he has a case of pneumonia. Generally, they said, this would not be a problem but it is exacerbated by the cancer which has weakened his immune system. I don't know much more than that. I'm booked on the overnight flight leaving this evening and I'm not sure exactly when I'll be back. I know you can't offer any technical advice, but I sure appreciate being able to talk to you about it."

"I'll be blunt," said Joe. "This does not sound like good news. Most of the people I see and meet are dealing with cancers that have not spread, but once they do, the options are considerably more limited. The best that we can hope for now is that Dennis is able to fight off the pneumonia. If not, we should pray for him to be comfortable. Please express to Barbara that I'm thinking of them both. Call me when you get back and let me know how things are going."

"I'll do that. Right now I need to run to one last meeting and then go home and pack. I sure wish you were here to help me get to the airport."

After they hung up Joe thought of calling Maria again, but checked his watch and realized that Maria would have already left for work.

He ate a light supper and tried watching television but he couldn't put Dennis out of his mind. Or Barbara and Bill. Finally he went to bed, but he couldn't fall asleep. He thought about Mr. Ruiz and Dennis and about his own situation. He realized that both Mr. Ruiz and Dennis had cancer that had probably started long before Joe's, and that in both cases had progressed much farther. But he also realized that, but for the grace of God, he could be in a similar situation in just a few years.

He went to sleep being thankful that his doctor was attentive to his lab test results. He had heard of doctors who ignored elevated PSA levels.

A few days later was another holiday. This was Hangeul Proclamation Day, which commemorates the invention (1443) and the proclamation (1446) of Hangeul, the native alphabet of the Korean language. Koreans are proud that Hangeul is a very scientific and creative artificial alphabet, and that it is one of the most recent official writing systems ever created. King Sejong the Great, inventor of Hangeul, is the most honored ruler in Korean history. This is a National Flag Raising Day and a National Celebration Day, but is not a Public Day Off, and the NCC was running on a regular schedule.

On Friday evening, Joe went with Mr. Morgan and Mr. Bailey to see a musical show called Jump. The show was a non-verbal performance packed with gymnastics, martial arts, and sight-gags. Joe was glad he didn't have to figure out what the performers were saying, since he wouldn't have been able to understand it. In a way, this show was like a very good version of Cirque de Soleil, as he had seen on television.

After the two holidays and the tour of Imjingak sandwiched in between, Joe was ready for something a little different. On the Saturday after his fifth week of treatment, Joe went to the Everland Theme Park. Joe had been to other theme parks, including Disney World in Florida, and generally knew what to expect. The park has three main sections called Festival World, Caribbean Bay, and Speedway. Festival World and Caribbean Bay have themed rides and performances. Speedway is an auto race track, offering traditional racing events. There is also a safari animal park where patrons can ride in special caged vehicles through an area with wild animals. Joe enjoyed himself, but felt a little guilty that he was having this much fun without his family.

Sunday was rainy and chilly, so Joe slept in, then went to A TwoSome Place and got a newspaper and some coffee. Later he watched some movies at his apartment, streaming the movies from Netflix.

When Joe called Maria on Sunday evening, she told him that Bill was back from Miami and would like to speak to Joe.

"He said to call Sunday morning at any time. He will be up early."

Joe knew Bill's home number and called as soon as he and Maria were finished talking.

Bill answered. "Joe, I knew it was you. I let Rosario sleep in and I came in here to make some coffee. I got back yesterday morning. Dennis is stable but he will be in the hospital for several days until the pneumonia is taken care of. I spent most of the time talking to Barbara since Dennis was only awake briefly from time to time. I think Barbara is starting to understand the inevitable. It's sure tough on her. How are you doing?"

Joe wasn't exactly ready for the shift in conversation.

"I'm doing well. I've had five weeks of treatment and have three more scheduled. And I've had the opportunity to visit many wonderful and exciting places here in Korea. I really want to come back here again with Maria and the girls. This is a great place to visit. But enough of me; I'm fine. Let's get back to your situation. How are you holding up?"

"Well I'm okay. Dennis is a good friend and I've known him and Barbara a long time. We can all wish things had been different. Comparing your case with Dennis' I can see now that if Dennis had responded a little differently he wouldn't be in this situation. Now I can only hope that he is comfortable and my attention has turned to trying to help Barbara cope."

They talked a little more about Joe's treatment. Except for the two times this week, Joe had not spoken with Bill since he had arrived in Korea. They agreed that Bill would keep Joe updated on the situation.

Joe wished Bill well and told him to pass on to Barbara his concern.

After his sixth week Joe realized that he was on the downhill side of his time in Korea and reviewed his notes to make sure he got to all the places he really wanted to see. He decided that snow or no snow, he should go to Pyeongchang to see where the 2018 Winter Olympics were to take place.

On Saturday morning, Joe traveled to Pyeongchang by train, a distance of just over 100 miles from Seoul. Joe found out that this route would be served by a KTX high-speed train in time for the 2018 Winter Olympics. The area is mountainous and is attractive in warmer months for such activities as fishing, whitewater rafting, hiking, as well as the beautiful views. A principal attraction in the winter are various winter sports.

Joe learned that in addition to the sports facilities, the community was making other preparations for the Olympics, such as setting up a marketing initiative known as The Best of Korea, which is designed to give a high quality experience to visitors from around the world.

Joe returned on Sunday afternoon, again loaded with photographs to send to Teresa.

On Thursday evening during Joe's regular call to Maria, she said, "Bill called last night. He said to tell you that Dennis' pneumonia had cleared up sufficiently to allow him to be moved to hospice."

"Hospice?" said Joe, a little startled. "Not a nursing home? That must mean that they think the things are worse than I thought. Okay, thanks. I'll try to get Bill at his office."

Joe called Bill, who answered quickly.

"I told Maria that you didn't need to call."

"I know," said Joe. "I am just concerned about how Dennis is getting on. Going to hospice seems like the end is inevitable."

"It is. I think we are all resolved now to simply wait it out and hope Dennis is comfortable. Even Barbara seems to be handling it. I promise to let you know if there is any change. When do you return?"

"In about three weeks. I'll have Maria let you know the details as soon as I have them."

"Okay, and I will let you know if anything happens."

Again Joe went to sleep wondering about how things could have been and was glad that he was nearing the end of his journey on a more positive note.

For his last weekend outing before returning to Argentina, Joe chose to take a little longer trip to Jinju in south-central Korea. The area is noted for its educational institutions and culture. The trip took several hours, so Joe left Friday afternoon, taking the KTX high-speed train to Busan and connecting with a local train to Jinju. This gave him all day Saturday to see the sights and allowed him to leave after breakfast on Sunday so he had plenty of time to get back to Seoul. Joe came to Jinju too late to experience the Namgang Lantern Festival that is held earlier in October, with the spectacle of lanterns floating down the Nam River. But he did have the opportunity to sample some of the region's cuisine.

Joe began his last week of treatment on a high note. He was starting to get excited about completing the treatment, which was going very well. More than that he was starting to be really excited to get home and be with Maria and the girls. He did realize, however, that he was going to miss the unique culture of Korea and especially the people he had come to genuinely appreciate.

On Tuesday the National Cancer Center put on a graduation for Joe and the other members of his class: Mr. Morgan and Mr. Bailey. They had cake and punch and had the chance to say goodbye to some of the staff they didn't see every day. Joe noted that while many of the staff probably went to one of these parties nearly every week, they still were genuine in their affection for the patients and truly regretted their having to leave.

Joe and the other two shared a taxi back to the apartment and decided on the way to go out for a round of soju. The bar they went to was not exceptionally busy, so they were able to talk easily. Their discussion concerned their experiences in Seoul and eventually turned to their disease and the satisfaction they shared with the treatment they received at the NCC.

After one round, Joe returned to his apartment and made his regular call to Maria.

Finally, it came time for Joe's adventure in Korea to end. Tests showed no sign of his tumor. He would need to take follow-up tests, including a PSA test every three months to track his progress. For the rest of his life Joe would have to get tested and monitor his situation.

On his last day at the NCC Joe had to deal with his discharge paperwork. Before leaving he sought out and thanked several of the doctors and staff for their contributions to his treatment. He promised to email them to let them know how he and the family were doing.

When the weekend came and Joe's treatments had ended, he turned his attention to packing and preparing to leave. He took a local trip to Insa-dong to pick up some interesting looking traditional Korean dresses for the girls, Maria, and Rosario. He also picked up a miniature desk-top Korean warrior figure in full battle dress for Bill to put on his desk at work.

Joe decided to pack and ship the various gifts along with some of his clothes and other gear rather than attempting to carry them in his luggage. Wendy assisted him in finding packing materials and arranging for the shipment at UPS.

Joe took a taxi with his shipment to UPS and then returned to the DMC Ville by subway. As he came into the lobby, he ran into Mr. Morgan and Mr. Bailey who had also graduated and were also getting ready to leave town.

"Come on, Joe, let's go celebrate our new credentials."

Joe joined them at a local tavern for a round of soju but begged off an extended evening of partying.

"I will be leaving tomorrow and need to finish packing tonight and get up early to make the plane."

"We're not leaving for a couple more days," said Mr. Morgan. "We're going to have a little fun."

"Righto," added Mr. Bailey. "Tomorrow morning we don't have to drink a gallon or two of water."

"Hear, hear." They toasted their new status.

When Joe returned to his apartment he packed his gear and then placed his regular call to Maria.

"Well, I leave tomorrow and this is our last call. I'll need to find a pay phone when I'm in Atlanta changing planes. I am really looking forward to getting back and being able to actually hug you and the girls, rather than just look at images on a computer screen."

"We're looking forward to having you back," Maria said in a somber tone.

"Why, what's the matter, Maria?" Joe picked up on her tone.

"Bill called a few minutes ago. Dennis has taken a turn for the worse at the hospice and Bill is leaving this evening to go up there. He said to let you know that he would be gone, so he will have to put off welcoming you back. He didn't sound happy."

"Oh boy," Joe thought to himself. He had been prepared for this, but it still came as a shock.

The next day was the big day. Joe was escorted to the airport by Wendy, who was also to meet a new arrival. Joe's return trip took a reverse route from his earlier journey but, due to the time change, he arrived in Atlanta shortly before he left Korea, and connected with his flight to Buenos Aries. The flight was overnight, and he arrived early the next morning.

Joe had only imagined how happy he would be to see Maria and the girls, but the emotion exceeded even his expectations. Not only was he seeing them after his longest separation from them ever, he was seeing them after having confronted a dreaded disease.

Websites Joe used to plan and carry out his Korea experience

Note: for updated information on websites and other information in this book, please see www.RoadToNamiIsland.blogspot.com.

Korea Tourism Organization (KTO) - This is the website for the official tourist organization of the Korean government, and has many useful links, including tour packages, visa and customs information, currency exchange information, etc. - http://asiaenglish.visitkorea.or.kr/ena/index.kto

National Cancer Center (NCC) - www.ncc.re.kr/english/proton/introduction.jsp

KMI International - The organization that facilitates medical tourism in Korea. - http://www.internationalkmi.com/

Blog created to assist American and Canadian teachers who travel to Korea as teachers of English - http://thedailykimchi.blogspot.com/

DMC Ville - The serviced apartment where foreign NCC patients stay. - http://www.dmcville.co.kr/

Seoul subway map -
http://www.nsubway.co.kr/korea/seoul/seoulsubwaymapen.htm

Seoul City Bus Tour -
http://en.seoulcitybus.com/sub.php?PN=introduction_sctb&mainNum=1&
subNum=11

English language newspapers published in Korea:
Korea Times - http://www.koreatimes.co.kr/www/index.asp
Korea Herald - http://www.koreaherald.com/
Korea JoongAng Daily - http://joongangdaily.joins.com/

Korea Train Express (KTX) - The high-speed passenger train system
providing access to many parts of Korea. Links here explain fares, timetables,
and special passes. - http://en.wikipedia.org/wiki/KTX and
http://info.korail.com/2007/eng/eng_index.jsp

Itaewon Shopping District -
http://visitkorea.or.kr/enu/SH/SH_EN_7_2_6_1.jsp

North Seoul Tower - http://en.wikipedia.org/wiki/N_Seoul_Tower

Football Club Seoul (soccer) - http://en.wikipedia.org/wiki/FC_Seoul

Jinju Lantern Festival - http://vimeo.com/29962935

Insadong - http://visitkorea.or.kr/enu/SH/SH_EN_7_2_2_1.jsp

Pyeongchang -
http://english.visitkorea.or.kr/enu/SI/SI_EN_3_1_1_1.jsp?cid=1351776

CHAPTER 7. TOO LATE

Joe's arrival in Buenos Aires was like that of a soldier returning home from the front. He took an overnight flight from Atlanta and arrived early the next morning. Maria had taken off work and the girls had taken off from school that morning to come meet him. He felt a rush of affection for them. After the hugging and kissing, they gathered his bags and went home.

"It's funny," said Joe. "When I traveled from Atlanta to Seoul I left one day and got there the next, but the sun was up for the entire trip. When I went the other direction, from Seoul to Atlanta, I went through a night and it was night most of the way, but I arrived in Atlanta before I left Seoul."

The girls giggled.

"We're not going to believe that one until we work it out," said Teresa.

"When you figure it out, I hope you'll understand why I may be off a little for a few days and won't be sure what day it is."

Guessing (correctly) that he had not eaten, Maria had made a breakfast casserole that was staying warm in the oven, so when they got home they all ate together. The girls left after that to go to school for the rest of the day.

"Well, let's see," said Joe, "I haven't spoken with you since I called from Atlanta late yesterday afternoon before I had to get ready for my flight. Is there any news?"

He meant this to be jovial, alluding to the fact that they had kept in close touch during the entire time he was away.

"In fact there is," said Maria somberly. "Rosario called last night shortly after you and I talked. Bill left Tuesday night and got to Miami yesterday morning and went straight to the hospice. Barbara was there and had been crying. Dennis was having a relapse and wasn't doing well, but he woke up long enough to recognize Bill. Bill was able to talk to Dennis briefly. Dennis asked Bill to make sure Barbara was cared for. Bill and Barbara stayed with Dennis but he didn't wake up again and died that afternoon."

"Rosario said that when he left, Bill had expected to return by this weekend or early next week as he had in his previous trips. Instead, he has to stay a few extra days to help Barbara with arrangements and to attend the funeral. Rosario says he is going to want to get with you as soon as he can after he gets back."

Joe absorbed all this slowly. The various messages and brief discussions with Bill over the last few weeks gave him a pretty clear idea of where things were headed, but when it happens you're never completely prepared. He would definitely meet with Bill.

"The situation with Dennis really brings me back to reality," he said. "All this time, I feel like I have been leading a charmed life. I found out that I had cancer; I discovered what I believe was the right solution; my treatment appears to have been successful; and I have a positive attitude about my prognosis. Still, I have nagging worries that something will go wrong. And I can't shake the fact that, but for a couple of lucky breaks, my story might have turned out like Dennis' story. I could have missed my physical. The doctor could have omitted the PSA test - remember the digital exam didn't show anything unusual. The doctor could have played down the extent and the seriousness of the disease, as did Dennis' doctor. I could have delayed the biopsy and the treatment. I could have taken the urologist's recommendation and accepted surgery, which might have left some cancer cells behind. My cancer was apparently not as far along as Dennis, but it could have progressed at a different rate. It could just as easily have been me suffering the fate Dennis suffered. And it could have just as easily been you and girls who would be in the position that Barbara is in now."

He turned away so Maria wouldn't see the tear forming in the corner of his eye.

Maria understood Joe. She put a hand on his arm and put her other arm over his shoulders.

"I understand you," she said. Neither one said anything more for a few minutes, and then Maria continued. "I understand you. We all have to live with hope, however. After all, there are several important differences between what happened to Dennis and what happened to you. You took charge of your situation as soon as you found out that there might be a problem. You didn't rely solely on what the doctor said. You did your own research and investigation. You found the option of proton therapy. You found the National Cancer Center in Seoul. No one handed you this information and found the solutions for you. You did it, and when you found out some important piece of information, you discussed it with the doctors. And I'm proud of you."

Joe realized she was right, and it helped clear things up in his own mind. His next question to himself was "what can I do with what I have learned?"

Joe had left cooler weather in Korea, turning from early fall toward winter. He returned to Buenos Aires with the weather turning from early spring toward summer. He spent most of the next few days with Maria and the girls. They went to the park and had picnics and enjoyed each other's company and the beautiful weather. But school was still in session, and Joe needed to get back to his office.

Through the wonders of the Internet and global communications, he had been able to make some use of the business center at DMC Ville, the apartment complex where he stayed, and had been able to keep up with his clients. The report analyzing the site for the large industrial complex had been accepted and the client was anxious to have Joe evaluate another project. An attorney had contacted him about preparing to testify in a civil case between a contractor and a builder concerning the detrimental impact of an unauthorized change to a design, but he had found it necessary to refer that project to one of his competitors as he would not return in time to undertake the task. He did, however, receive a couple of smaller projects that he was able to complete remotely with the help of his assistant.

So after a few days spent with the family, Joe went into the office and in a couple of days brought everything current. He also scheduled a trip to meet with the client who wanted him to undertake the new project.

As soon as Bill returned from Miami, he and Joe arranged for lunch at the restaurant near the tennis club and agreed to meet a little later so they would be able to linger, if necessary in order to complete their conversation.

Bill and Joe arrived at almost the same time and were shown to a table near the windows. Unlike the scene a few months before, this time the garden was in full flower and the grass was green and fresh. A few late diners were finishing their lunch at the tables outside on the patio, but Bill and Joe elected to stay inside.

Bill summarized the situation as soon as they had ordered. "As you know, I made several trips to Miami over the last couple of months. I think the clerks at the airline were beginning to recognize me. I know I kept you up to date while you were gone, but let me set the stage by repeating some of the story. As you recall, Dennis had surgery at the beginning of this year. Within a few months, it was obvious that the surgery had not removed all his cancer. In addition, it became obvious that his cancer had spread to his lymph nodes. From there it moved quickly to his bones and throughout his body. He began hormone treatments shortly after my first trip to Miami, before you left for Korea. The treatments were a matter of too little, too late. The doctors added hormone treatments to try to stop the growth of the cancer, but that didn't work."

"While you were in Korea, Dennis kept getting worse. When he had trouble breathing Barbara had to call an ambulance. They took him to the hospital and determined that he had pneumonia. He stayed in the hospital for several days until his condition improved. At that point the doctors recommended that Barbara put him in hospice. I think that was the toughest part for her because it confirmed again that Dennis' condition was terminal. I think she expected to take him home where he could recover and things would return to normal, to the extent that things had been normal."

"I got there just after Dennis was moved to hospice. I had seen him at the hospital, and I must say that he was much better looking and seemed to be in better shape at the hospice. But of course he had to improve from the bout of pneumonia before he could even be moved to hospice. His appearance was on the surface only. In the meantime his cancer was eating away at him. But his death wasn't any less shocking."

"It was a nasty business," Bill concluded. "Dennis had lost a lot of weight and was clearly not his normal, animated self. They gave him drugs to ease the pain. It was not good. And as bad as it obviously was for Dennis, it is worse for Barbara. Dennis was finally able to escape his misery, but she has to continue to live with it."

"Incidentally, Barbara was floored by how hospice was handling Dennis' case. When he was admitted she had to sign papers and found out that they would not be giving him any medicine to help him get well but would simply attempt to make him comfortable and help him avoid undue pain. They described it to her as letting his body go through the process of shutting down. Actually, I think that helped her close the door on any notion that Dennis' death was not inevitable."

Bill was very somber and they both ate silently. Neither was very hungry, and they left most of their meals.

"I hope I don't have to remind you to have your PSA tested regularly," said Joe as he pushed his plate aside and took a sip of coffee.

Bill chuckled at what was close to graveyard humor. "Oh I have learned that lesson, believe me."

Joe sat back in his seat.

"This situation with Dennis has been tough on you," said Joe, "and tough on everyone you love, I know. And it has been especially bad on Barbara. I know that, too. That's maybe too obvious to even say. But you have to step back a little and take a larger view. Things happen to people. Some are good, and some are bad. Some things a person can control, and some things a person can't control. Some things a person could control but doesn't. Sometimes, a person would exercise some control if he knew what to do but either doesn't know or chooses not to try to influence the outcome."

"In my own humble opinion, Dennis got bad advice up and down the line. That wasn't his fault, but the lesson is that you need to go beyond the advice you get and find out as much as you can for yourself. That might or might not have changed things with Dennis, but it's the way things happened. It didn't work out for him. It's sad, but the question for us is what do we do about it?"

"While I was in Korea, I ran into a number of situations and heard a number of stories. Some had good outcomes and some didn't."

"For example, I met some men at the National Cancer Center who were having what they call salvage radiation treatment at the proton facility. These men had surgery before, but the surgery had not been successful in removing all the cancer, so they had proton therapy to remove what was left. This is not possible in all cases. Proton beam therapy cannot be used in the cancer has spread beyond the prostate itself. Apparently Dennis' situation would not have qualified since the cancer had apparently already spread.

"I heard another story which was, in some ways similar to Dennis' story. This was the case of a man in his 70s, who led an active lifestyle and had a somewhat younger wife. He was diagnosed with prostate cancer and was advised by his urologist to have surgery. He had a friend who told him about proton therapy and who helped him search out information on proton. He apparently knew as much about the choices of the different forms of treatment as I knew after I did my research. This included knowing about the side effects of the different forms of treatment. Despite all this, he chose to have the surgery. Afterwards, he came to find out that he would be suffering the side effects, basically for the rest of his life. The side effects of loss of bladder control hampered his active lifestyle, and his younger wife was not happy that he lost his ability to achieve an erection.

"I saw or heard about a number of cases that were apparently the result of delays in pursuing any form of proactive treatment. There are few signs of prostate cancer and those signs are very subtle. Men can have cancers that are evolving and spreading without any indication that any kind of a problem is occurring. The notion that the disease is slow to develop avoids the reality that it does, in fact, develop. When there are delays in treatment the prospects to achieving success decrease, particularly when it comes to long-term success.

"When it comes down to it," concluded Joe, "men need to make sure they are getting PSA tests and they need to make sure their doctors are carefully considering the results. They need to ask questions and become aware of their own situations."

"So what's next in the Dennis story?" asked Joe, changing the focus a little.

"When I left after the funeral, Barbara was leaving to spend a couple of weeks with a cousin in her home town. Barbara has a degree in elementary education, but she never worked while Dennis was alive. I think her plan is to update her credentials, get a teaching certificate, and start teaching. I think her cousin is a teacher and told her they have opportunities in the local school system there. I'll be going up in a couple of weeks to help her with arranging the sale of their house and moving out."

They talked a little longer about other things, and then decided that it was time to leave. The restaurant was empty and the tables were being prepared for dinner. They agreed to keep each other posted.

"We're getting on toward Christmas," commented Joe. "I sure hope things become more merry from here on."

"I agree," replied Bill.

Joe headed home as his work for the day was finished. He decided to walk due to the nice weather.

That evening Maria had another planning committee meeting for the tennis tournament and the girls had a club meeting to attend, so Joe made a sandwich and retired to the home office to ponder.

While he was in Korea Joe had met many people and heard many stories. As his treatment progressed, he became less centered on his own situation and started to be more aware of the situations others were going through.

On a whim, Joe went on his computer and checked on a couple of the blogs maintained by former prostate patients. Earlier, during his research he had used these as sources of information on different forms of treatment. The information was particularly helpful because it reflected the personal experiences of actual patients. While it was not scientific research, the large number of men who posted their own stories helped him understand some of the patterns.

As an example, Joe quickly got the sense that not all doctors were aware of proton beam therapy to the extent that he felt they needed to be. Also, many men indicated that the doctors they initially approached were focused on recommending treatments that were the ones they themselves delivered; radiation oncologists recommended radiation, surgeons recommended surgery, and so forth. These bits of information helped Joe understand the overall situation better and warned him to question and check on some of the information he was given.

After being treated, however, Joe realized that there were many other valuable uses for the blogs. He noticed that in posting their stories, men were helping others understand the side effects of their treatment. In cases where men were suffering side effects they could not avoid, the blog posts helped them cope with their situation.

The blogs also created a forum for men to share ideas and even to advocate positions. A recent example was the reaction to suggestions in the United States that PSA testing be undertaken in a more limited manner, as opposed to promoting it for more men. Joe realized that if it weren't for the PSA testing he would be completely oblivious to his disease and could be on a path to suffer Dennis' fate.

When Maria got home he sat with her in the living room while they waited up for the girls.

Joe told Maria all about his lunch with Bill and the Dennis story.

"I really feel for Barbara," Maria said. "I occasionally find myself wondering what it would have been like for me and the girls if you were the one in the situation Dennis found himself in. Thanks goodness they didn't have children. I hope Barbara is able to get on her feet and doesn't have to suffer too much emotionally as a result of this."

"I have come across a number of blogs that describe support groups that could help," answered Joe. "I'll get some of the information and give it to Bill to send to her."

"Good idea."

"Do you recall that while we were doing our research I mentioned that it might be nice to talk to some of the men who were posting on these blogs? You know, actually talk to them on the phone."

"I remember that. You never did, although you read many of their posts."

"When it came to the point where I discovered a lot of that information I had already largely settled on proton beam therapy in Korea and I thought that my questions were already being answered. Now I see that there are many useful benefits of staying in touch with these people after treatment. There is still a lot of knowledge that is needed, and I expect to be around for a good many years.

"You know the situation with Dennis will always influence how I look back on my own experience. When someone who has to face a problem has a completely different outcome as compared with someone else with essentially the same problem, you have to ask why each had the outcome he had and not the alternative outcome. I keep coming back to the fact that it could just as well have been me."

"I understand," said Maria, "but sometimes you have to put it aside and move ahead rather than try to analyze it too much. Maybe you can focus your energy on figuring out ways to share the information you have learned with others so that it can be useful to them."

"Excellent point."

Joe placed a call to Bill.

"I have some information on support groups for prostate patients and their loved ones. I'll gather it up and send it to you and you can send it on to Barbara. Will you do that?"

"Excellent idea," said Bill. "I hadn't thought about that, but it may be useful."

CHAPTER 8. PROTON BEAM THERAPY AND OTHER CANCERS

A couple of weeks before Christmas, Joe and Maria attended a Christmas party at the tennis club with Bill and Rosario. Soon after they arrived, they were having a glass of wine when a friend of the two women came up to greet them. While engaging in chit-chat, the woman happened to mention another family they all knew.

"Did you hear that the Garzas took their son to the doctor? He had been having some kind of seizures and they didn't know what was wrong. The doctors couldn't tell at first what was happening. Finally they had an MRI done and discovered a tumor near his spine, just below his brain. The operated on the tumor but couldn't get all of it because of its location. They are worried about using traditional x-rays because of the potential long term damage from radiation on the brain and spinal cord."

"Really," exclaimed Joe. This was the first time he had known anyone who had a child afflicted by cancer. He had known the Garzas for several years, although not nearly as well as Maria had.

He glanced at Maria, realizing she would be more in shock than he was. She was just staring at the woman and gripping Rosario's arm. Rosario was staring, too. Joe figured he needed to check everyone, so he glanced at Bill. Bill was intently listening but did not appear to be in shock. Bill knew the Garzas about as well as Joe did.

Changing the subject slightly, Joe asked "Who is their doctor?" He wasn't exactly sure why he asked the question, but it came out.

"Doctor Silva," said the woman. "He's your family doctor, too, isn't he?"

"Why, yes he is." Joe began to think.

Something had come to Joe's attention while he was researching alternative prostate cancer treatments and later while he was in Korea. He learned that proton beam therapy can be used for treating a variety of cancers other than prostate cancer. At the time, Joe was very much focused on his own prostate cancer, however, and he paid little attention to this knowledge.

After he returned from Korea, the possibilities for using proton beam therapy increasingly became a part of his thoughts. What he had learned initially and through further study on the Internet was that several cancers lend themselves to use of this therapy, including lung cancer, cancer of the eye and brain, and a number of pediatric cancers. Big news among those interested in proton therapy was that it had been recently approved in the United States for use in treatment of breast cancers.

Not being an oncologist of course, Joe only had a general notion of what made a pediatric cancer case a good candidate for proton treatment. It appeared to him as a layman that there were two reasons, both resulting from the fact that more precise aiming of the beam allowed delivery of a higher dose with reduced impact on adjacent healthy cells.

First, certain cancers are located in places in the body very close to sensitive organs, such as the heart and brain. In these locations, stray radiation from x-rays would not just do damage to healthy tissue, but would damage very sensitive healthy tissue. The more precise aiming of the proton beam allows the beam to be brought closer to the targeted cancer cells with less collateral damage to adjoining tissues.

Second, children have growing bodies and are more susceptible to radiation-caused diseases and tissue damage. If the beam can be aimed more precisely and less collateral damage done, the child would suffer fewer side effects. Among children this was really important, as the side effects have been shown to impair normal physical development of the body, as well as impair mental growth.

Joe also knew that traditional radiation can induce additional cancers that weren't there to begin with. He wondered if this might be exacerbated in the more sensitive tissues of young children.

The kinds of cancers that cannot be treated with proton beam therapy are those that are distributed throughout the body, such as cancers of the blood, or cancers that have metastasized, meaning that are no longer confined to their initial location but have spread out to other parts of the body. One issue that is always of concern to prostate cancer patients is to get treatment before the disease spreads into the lymph nodes, from which it can spread to other parts of the body.

To a large extent, this information was academic to Joe, as he had no particular way of using it.

"Maybe until now," he thought to himself.

The rest of the evening went by in a daze for Maria and Rosario, with Joe and Bill focused on shepherding their wives through the protocol. It was traditional at this annual event for everyone to gather around a grand piano in the ballroom and sing a couple of Christmas carols. As soon as that was accomplished, it was no longer impolite to leave, and Joe suggested that they go. The others agreed.

As they waited at the porte-cochere for the valet to return their cars, Joe said "I know this situation with the Garza boy is something of a shock. We're adults, however, and instead of fretting about it, let's see if there is something we can actually do about it."

"What could we possibly do?" asked Rosario.

"Well, I don't really know. But I do know from my own recent experience that there is more information to be gathered and I think we could turn our attention to that task."

Maria and Rosario looked more relieved all of a sudden.

"To start with," continued Joe, "let's hit the Internet. Also, I'll pay a visit to Doctor Silva tomorrow. I owe him a visit. I called him when I returned last month, but he wasn't available and I haven't gotten around to calling him again. I'll talk to him and see if I can find out more about the type of condition the boy has. I suspect that it's not ethical for him to talk about the specific case, but I can find out more about this type of case in general."

The valet brought Bill's car and the friends said goodnight.

"I'll help with the Internet searches," said Maria. "I got pretty good at that when I was helping you before."

For the first time since she heard the news earlier in the evening, a hint of a smile came across her face.

Their car came, and they got in and drove home. Both were thinking.

The girls had just finished exams that day. The next day would be Thursday and would be the last day of school until it resumed in March following the summer vacation. School closed a day early because many families set out on vacation trips on Friday. Joe had often explained to the girls that when they moved to the United States, they would have their summer vacation in the middle of the year because the summer season in the Northern Hemisphere is the opposite of summer season south of the Equator.

They greeted Joe and Maria with big hugs.

"I guess the thrill of completing the school year is in your hearts," said Maria. Joe chuckled.

"Yes, it's a great feeling," said Teresa, "and we just got to see our favorite singer on television. Now I'm tired."

"Me too," said Victoria. The girls headed for their room and bed.

"I'm going to look at a couple of things on the computer and check my email," Joe told Maria, "but there's not much point in getting heavily into this new project until I get more information from Doctor Silva."

Joe changed for bed, then went into the home office and messed briefly with the computer. When he got back to the bedroom, Maria was in bed and reading a book.

"It would be a good thing if we could actually find something that could help the Garzas," she said, putting the book down.

Joe flipped off the light and snuggled into bed, wrapping his arm around Maria. She snuggled up to him.

"I'm interested," she said with a slight giggle. "I don't know if you've noticed, but ever since you returned from Korea, sex has been better."

"I have noticed."

The next morning, Joe left early for the office. As soon as he got there, he placed a call to Doctor Silva's office and asked if the doctor was in.

"The doctor is not in yet," said his receptionist, "but his schedule is pretty light today. Would you care to see him?"

"Yes I would, but this is mostly a social visit, not a medical appointment."

"In that case, can you come right now? His first official appointment is not until ten."

"I'll be right there," said Joe.

When he got to the doctor's office, the doctor had just arrived.

"Why, Joe! What a surprise. What brings you here? I hope there is nothing wrong," the doctor said, ending with a slight frown.

"Oh, no," said Joe. "I have some questions and I realized I hadn't seen you since I got back. I called, but with one thing and another either you were busy or I was busy."

The doctor ushered Joe into his office, asking his receptionist to bring them coffee.

"So, tell me all about it."

Joe gave a concise description of his trip to Korea, the treatments, and his exploration of Seoul and Korea. He could tell that the doctor had many questions, but he tried to hold the doctor off so he could get to the real point of his visit before his time ran out.

"I see we have a lot more to talk about and I know your time is limited this morning. Perhaps we could get together for lunch," said Joe, glancing at his watch. "Let me switch to another subject if I may. My wife and I were with some people at the tennis club last night and we heard about the Garza boy's cancer. I know you can't talk specifically about the case, but I would like some general information about children's cancers."

"Of course, as you say I cannot reveal details of this case but let me speak more generally," said Doctor Silva, becoming serious.

"It is always a sad thing with children with any disease. Children are so vulnerable and a disease such as cancer can so impair their very lives. Not only do they have to fight the disease, which takes them away from their normal activities like playing and going to school and socializing with other children, but both the disease and the treatment can affect their physical and mental growth. These diseases affect adults, too, but adults have usually achieved the full extent of their physical size and abilities and have grown mentally to the point where they will remain for life."

"What kinds of treatments are available?" asked Joe.

"Speaking generally, for diseases such as cancer the treatments are much the same as they are for adults, but the side effects can be greater. Typically, treatment of pediatric cancers include surgery to debulk the tumor, even if the entire tumor cannot be removed. In addition, some radiation and some chemotherapy are usually required.

"Gaining clear margins with surgery in a case like this will be very difficult because of the proximity of the tumor to the brain and spine meaning additional treatment will be necessary. As an example, for Ewing's Sarcoma there will be 17 rounds of chemotherapy required as it is treated as a systemic disease even though it was not thankfully metastatic when discovered. After approximately six rounds of chemotherapy, the child will be evaluated for additional surgery and a phase of radiation. The parents need to consider some form of conformal radiation treatment such as IMRT or, better yet, proton therapy.

"As I said before, the developing bodies of young children are more susceptible to the side effects resulting from these treatments. For example, children are more susceptible to radiation-induced sarcomas. Recent studies have shown that proton therapy has been shown to reduce this risk by from 25 to 50 percent. Also, traditional radiation in pediatric brain tumors has been associated with long-term neurocognitive deficits including decreases in IQ, difficulties with attention, processing speed and other executive skills. Also, even low dose radiation to glands in the brain may have a life-long detrimental effect on hormone production and growth. Protons have the ability to target tumors with high precision and have no exit dose.

"I of course referred this case to the best specialists in Argentina and they do not have a good, clear answer and are researching current protocols used on this disease so I can help advise them."

"Can you give me the medical name of the disease?" asked Joe.

"Well, yes, but what do you have in mind?" The doctor wrote the medical term on a pad and handed it to Joe. It said "Ewing's Sarcoma."

Joe had never heard of it.

"When I was in Korea I learned that there were a number of pediatric cancers being treated with proton beam therapy. I looked at the results of studies on the internet and found that this is a growing area of interest. Some proton facilities even wish to focus more of their attention on pediatric cancer cases. I thought I would see if I could use some of my new contacts to look into whether this case would be a possible candidate. I would like to help the Garzas, but I don't want to approach them and get their hopes up unnecessarily. I know from my own experience how well-meaning people can upset people by giving advice that is inappropriate or misleading. If there is a good, legitimate basis for looking into proton beam therapy, I want to help them as much as I can with making the right contacts."

"Okay," said Doctor Silva, still not quite sure. "I have known the Garzas many years. I brought their little boy into the world. If you can make some contacts and the Garzas agree, I will cooperate as much as I can."

Joe thanked the doctor and said he would get back in touch as soon as possible.

Joe went back to his office and cleaned up, making a few calls and signing some letters. He wanted to get home and start his research. He also wanted to email the doctors at the National Cancer Center in Korea, but it was still in the middle of the night there.

After he finished his most important work, he left for lunch and told his assistant that he would be back the next day. He was starting to notice a slight slowdown in work activity as many of his clients and the people he dealt with were shifting their attention to Christmas.

He got home and made a sandwich. The girls would not return home from their last day at school for two more hours and Maria was still at the school library.

Joe went in to the home office, booted up his computer, and started searching for information on Ewing's Sarcoma, the type of cancer Doctor Silva had written on the pad.

After visiting a few websites, Joe turned his attention to composing an email to the National Cancer Center in Korea. Joe felt like he knew the doctors at the NCC well enough to get a response to his questions. He had not communicated with any of the staff at the NCC since he had returned, with the exception of filling out a questionnaire he had been given when he left. His first post-treatment appointment was scheduled for three months after he returned, which was still almost two months away. He realized that he missed them more than he would have expected.

Then an idea came to him. While it would still be a few hours until it would be morning in Seoul when the doctors could read and respond to an email, the NCC's representative in the United States, Curtis Poling, was in the same time zone as Joe was. Joe had spoken to Mr. Poling on several occasions before he went to Korea. Also, he had met Mr. Poling in person while he was in Korea as Mr. Poling frequently traveled to Seoul as part of his duties. Finally, Mr. Poling had called Joe after his return to Buenos Aires to check on him and to ask if he was having any side effects or if he had any questions or comments regarding his treatment. He recalled that almost all his official interactions with the NCC had been by emails to Mr. Poling, who forwarded them to the NCC.

He placed a call to Poling and left a voicemail message, saying he had a question about pediatric cancer treatment with proton beam therapy. Then he returned to his research.

A short while later, Mr. Poling called him back.

"Hello, Joe," he said. "How are you holding up?"

"Hello. I'm doing fine. I still have almost two months until I go in for my first follow-up exam and PSA test, but I feel great. I don't seem to have any side effects. By the way, I've noticed that sex is better. Is this something I should have expected?"

"Well," Mr. Poling began with a chuckle. "We don't have any definitive clinical information, and I'm not aware of any studies being done, but I have heard that from a number of former proton patients. It may be a while before someone actually pursues a study, since there is so much else we are trying to establish."

"Actually, there is something else I want to ask you about." Joe proceeded to relay the story of the Garza boy and what he had learned so far.

"Do you think that if I contacted Dr. Cho about this it might be something that can be treated with proton beam therapy?"

"It could be. I know that the National Cancer Center and other proton centers have been treating an increasing number of pediatric cases. However, it would be one of the other doctors, probably not Dr. Cho. Let me suggest that I go ahead and send an initial email and relate to them what you have already told me. I will confirm with them what kinds of information they will need in order to judge whether they can handle this case. While they won't be able to make a determination until they review the records, I think it would be safe for you to go ahead and approach the parents. Nothing can proceed until the parents agree, and for that they need to get the information.

"I will send an email right now. The doctors there will be at work in a few hours and it will be Friday there. If I don't send it soon, they might not get it until Monday their time, which will be Sunday evening our time."

"Okay," said Joe. "I just needed to know if there was a possibility. I would still have to convince the doctors and the child's parents here to participate, and I am not in a position to tell them that there is any definite chance for a successful outcome, or even whether the National Cancer Center would be in a position to accept the case. It's something like a Catch-22."

Mr. Poling told him to talk to the Garza's and, if they agreed, to send the medical records to him to be forwarded to the NCC. He said that the National Cancer Center would review them carefully and get a response as quickly as possible.

After ending the call, Joe decided to change gears and approach the Garza family, so he called and got Mrs. Garza on the first ring. Joe introduced himself.

"Oh, yes. I know you from the tennis club," Mrs. Garza said. "Actually, I know your wife very well. We have served on some committees together over the last few years. What can I do for you?"

"Actually, it's what I hope I can do for you. I hope you will not take offense, but I heard about the situation with your son and I have some information that might be of help."

Joe proceeded to tell an abbreviated version of his own story, and then explained what he had found out from his brief research.

"In short," he continued, "I am aware that there is an emerging opportunity to treat certain childhood cancers with what is called proton beam therapy. This is a form of therapy that very precisely delivers a dose of proton radiation in such a way as to minimize collateral damage to nearby sensitive tissues."

Before he got much more out, Mrs. Garza cut him off.

"I don't mean to sound rude, but it happens that we are looking into all serious ideas for treatment for our son. We have had several discussions with Dr. Silva and with the oncologist Dr. Silva referred us to and he agrees that we should consider all possibilities. My husband is having another meeting with Dr. Silva at this moment to discuss what we have learned. For some of the possible forms of treatment, money is an issue. Proton beam therapy has been mentioned, but the doctors have told us that it is not available in South America, but only available in the United States and in a few other places. They also told us that it is very expensive.

"My husband has scheduled a meeting tomorrow with the executive committee of the tennis club in which he will ask about the possibility of a charity exhibition or tournament to help raise funds to help pay for the expense of any appropriate treatment we identify. I keep hoping for a miracle, but it seems right now that we have a long way to go."

Joe could hear the stress in her voice.

"I may be speaking out of turn," Joe said, "but what I would like to do, if it is okay with you, is to come by and see you and your husband and answer any questions you might have. Would you be okay if I did that?"

Mrs. Garza agreed that it would be better for Joe to talk to the Garzas together. They arranged to meet that evening.

Joe thought about the conversation and about the bigger scenario that was unfolding. He felt uncomfortable appearing to intruding into what was a very private and sensitive matter, but his own experience with cancer and proton beam therapy suggested that he needed to be somewhat aggressive in bringing proton's existence to the attention of those who might need it.

The girls and Maria arrived home shortly, and Joe told Maria about his conversations with the doctor, with Mr. Poling, and with Mrs. Garza. They all agreed to have sandwiches so that they would be able to get to the Garza's house on time.

Joe told Maria about his reluctance to intrude and how it conflicted with his desire to make sure the Garzas had the information they needed.

"Don't worry about it," Maria told him. "The Garzas are very nice people. I know Mrs. Garza fairly well and I think she is strong enough to not get emotional. She will take the information and use it if she can."

She patted Joe on the hand and added, "Now finish your sandwich so we can go. I'll go see if we have another bottle of the red wine we like."

When they arrived at the Garza home, Mr. Garza greeted them at the door, smiling, and invited them in.

"A smile," Joe thought to himself. "That's a good sign. I hope it's not too forced."

They sat in the living room and Mrs. Garza offered them coffee.

Joe didn't want to intrude and thought they ought to get right to the point, but as soon as they sat Maria and Mrs. Garza began chatting quietly. Joe relaxed a little and let his wife handle the conversation.

"Before we get into anything else, please tell me how you are doing," Maria asked Mrs. Garza.

"This whole situation is very stressful, as I expect you can appreciate. All kinds of people have gone out of their way to contact us; some I feel truly care, but some seem only to give us unsolicited advice or make comments that are insensitive. I don't think they even realize it. When the next person tells me that things aren't as bad as they seem, I may want to punch them in the mouth. It is as bad as it seems; in fact, it's worse. I feel a little more comfortable talking to you two because I know you have just been through this and are probably sensitive to what others say."

Joe's sense of caution rose quickly at the mention of unsolicited advice, but settled back down as Mrs. Garza proceeded.

"I understand perfectly," he said. "I, too, had to listen to comments that were meant to be helpful and supportive but were truly insensitive. But this conversation is not about me, it's about your situation and your son's health. Please stop me if I am not helping, and understand that I don't like this kind of conversation, but I feel compelled to provide you with the benefit of my experience."

"We understand perfectly," said Mr. Garza, who had been quiet up to this point. "Let's go ahead and hear what you have and see what we can do with it."

Joe ran through the basics of cancer and the different therapies. He reviewed the kinds of side effects that are experienced from the different treatments, referring to websites and reports for substantiation. He explained that some pediatric cancers, in particular, were indicated for proton beam therapy. He explained in very brief terms about the characteristics of proton beam treatment that resulted in higher accuracy and reduced impact on surrounding healthy tissue.

"I'll forward to you a report I read that shows the statistics on the incidence of adverse side effects of proton beam therapy. It shows that in the case of pediatric cancers, adverse side effects are either negligible or are substantially lower than they are with other treatments.

"I should also warn you that this treatment may not be appropriate for your son. There are certain situations where proton beam therapy is not indicated, including cases where the cancer has spread. If you choose to pursue this course of action, you will need to forward your son's medical records to the proton center so they can evaluate the situation and determine if proton beam therapy can be used."

"That's all very helpful," said Mr. Garza when Joe had finished. "At the suggestion of Dr. Silva, I did have a brief discussion on proton therapy with the oncologist. Dr. Silva mentioned that you had received this treatment for your prostate cancer and told me this morning that you had discussed it with him. The oncologist said he had some limited familiarity with proton treatment but said there are no facilities in Argentina, or for that matter in South America. He suggested that we might pursue treatment in the United States where there are a number of such facilities.

"I must tell you, however, that cost is an issue. The oncologist had some information on that, and it does appear that this could be a major hurdle. We have been on the phone with various relatives seeing what kind of financial support we can get. Also, the national healthcare plan is reluctant to finance treatment outside the country, even when it is not available locally. Their position is that other forms of permitted treatment are available here. Based on what the oncologist was able to learn, we can come up with only about half of what the cost will be, which includes the cost of the treatment itself, along with the cost of transportation and housing at the treatment facility. You are aware that I plan to meet with the executive committee of the tennis club to discuss holding a tennis exhibition or tournament to try to help raise funds. This was a very difficult thing to do. I would really feel much better if it turned out that I wouldn't have to grovel like that."

Mr. Garza shrugged in desperation, and Joe detected a tear swelling in the corner of his eye.

"I may have a suggestion on that point," Joe said slowly. "As to the national health care, you may not be aware, but I am not a citizen of Argentina. Accordingly, I am not covered by the plan. I have private insurance but it is a relatively limited policy. When I discussed proton beam therapy with my insurance company, they agreed to pay the equivalent of what treatment would cost here and I was responsible for the balance. Perhaps the national healthcare would make a similar arrangement for you."

"Thanks, I'll look into that," said Mr. Garza.

"In addition, you need to understand that one of the reasons I chose to get treated in Korea was that the cost was substantially lower than it would have been in the United States. Also, the cost of treatment in Korea includes housing for the time you need to be there. You would be responsible only for getting to Korea, along with your food and incidental expenses."

"Well, that also sounds good. I'll look into that," added Mr. Garza. "What are my next steps to pursue this approach?"

"This is Thursday night. It's Friday morning in Korea. You need to contact both Dr. Silva and the oncologist and have your son's medical records forwarded to Mr. Curtis Poling in the United States. He is the representative for a company called KMI, which is responsible for marketing to the National Cancer Center in Seoul. Mr. Poling will advise as to exactly which records are needed, but I assume it will include any X-rays, CT scans, or MRI's, along with other detailed information about the cancer. A team of experts in Korea will review the records and make a determination as to whether or not your son is a candidate. The doctors can gather the records and they can be emailed tomorrow. If you need any help doing that, I can help. That would be soon enough because by the time they get to Korea it will be after business hours there. The records will be distributed and reviewed early next week, and unless they need more information or have some other questions, you should hear in a few days. If your son's case can be accepted you will be notified. At that time you will also get a cost estimate and some more information. Also, I should add that you will receive a treatment time sooner than would be the case at most American facilities."

"Okay. I'll follow up on this first thing in the morning. May I call you if I have any questions?"

"Certainly." Joe gave Mr. Garza his phone number at work and at home, along with his email address. "With your permission, I'll also forward your phone number and email address to Mr. Poling. He handles cases from around the world. He can also be very helpful, and he is in a time zone which is the same as ours. If you have any questions, call. I have a lunch meeting tomorrow, but otherwise I will be at one of those numbers."

"Well, we want to thank you both very much for this information. You know, we decided that we would need to listen to all ideas, even the crackpot ones if we were to have a chance to learn something useful. I'm very glad we heard from you."

Joe grinned. "I certainly support your reasoning on this. I don't know if I ever thought of proton beam therapy as a crackpot idea, but I was just as desperate as you are to find a solution. If it turns out to be appropriate for your son, I believe you will be pleased."

Both Mr. and Mrs. Garza seemed happier and more relieved than they had been when Joe and Maria had arrived. They all said their goodbyes and Joe and Maria left for home.

When they got home Joe went into the home office and checked his emails. Joe then sent a follow-up email to Curtis Poling bringing him up to date on the situation with the Garza boy and letting him know that he might be hearing from Mr. Garza soon. He also asked Mr. Poling if he knew what an approximate cost would be for this kind of treatment.

Maria made some coffee and she and Joe sat in the living room with the radio tuned to their favorite easy-listening station.

"I sure hope some good comes of this," Maria said. "The Garzas have some relatives who could help them, and it would be nice if the boy can be treated and the cost is within their reach. I know that is one of the things they are concerned about - the need to do something quickly."

"We'll keep our fingers crossed and pray that the medical information will allow this if it is the appropriate treatment, and that the cost issue works itself out," Joe responded. "There are still some difficulties with pediatric cases that are not found in treating adults. For one thing, small children, generally those under twelve years of age, have to be sedated in order to be treated, since they don't understand the need to be very still. I know this would be very difficult on the parents while the treatment is going on, but the potential outcome of overcoming the cancer is worth the anxiety and the frustrations they surely feel. Based on my research on the Internet, children who are treated with proton therapy don't suffer some of the consequences of radiation, including the loss of IQ and stunting of growth."

They each sat with their own thoughts.

The next day was Friday. While it was now the weekend in Korea, the Garza boy's doctors could be compiling the medical records to be sent to Mr. Poling and then to the NCC. The doctors at the NCC could begin their review next week. Joe hoped that Mr. Garza was not having any problems getting the information. When he and Maria had left the previous evening, he had told Mr. Garza to call him if there were any problems.

Joe was scheduled to meet with Bill for lunch. As usual, they had agreed to meet at the restaurant near the tennis club.

Bill arrived just after Joe was seated near the window overlooking the patio. Joe could tell that Bill was much more relaxed than he had been the last time they had met for lunch, when they had been discussing Dennis' death.

"I wonder why it seemed to be busy this week when it really wasn't," said Bill when he sat down.

"I think it's because there are lots of little things that need to be taken care of," responded Joe. "During regular times, those things get pushed off or handled quickly and more of our attention is on our bigger projects. With the bigger projects on hold, or at least on a slow speed, the little things become more apparent."

"I guess that explains it. Let's order."

After the waiter left, Bill started the conversation. "Tell me what you learned about the Garza boy."

Joe filled Bill in on his activities since the reception.

"I wasn't sure that the Garzas were going to be receptive to my suggestions, and I had to keep emphasizing that I was not trying to be a busybody. Thankfully they didn't seem unhappy that I approached them and are looking into the idea of pursuing proton therapy. Mr. Garza is checking with Dr. Silva and the oncologist today to get the medical records to forward to the NCC for review. I have emailed Mr. Poling, who is their representative in the United States to let them know that the records are coming. Of course it's now very early Saturday morning in Seoul and they won't be able to process the information for a couple of days. We'll just have to see how it works out."

Their meals arrived and they chatted a little more while they ate. Joe asked if Bill had heard anything from Barbara, Dennis' wife.

"Actually I have," said Bill. "As you know, I have been helping her wrap up Dennis' affairs, including selling the house. Barbara is going to move back to her hometown where she has a number of relatives. By the way, Barbara is a good friend of the women's tennis coach at the University of Miami. I told her at one point that your daughters, especially Teresa, are very good tennis players and Barbara happened to mention it to her friend. Now her friend, the coach, wants to find out more and wants to contact the coach at the girls' school. You may be looking at a scholarship or two in the future."

This news was a pleasant surprise for Joe. He would have to figure out a way to find out if the girls' coach had actually been contacted. He realized that he wasn't sure how these things worked.

After they ate, Bill got serious again.

"One more thing I'm curious about. I have been aware of proton therapy for prostate cancer as the result of your experience, but I realized I don't know that much about other diseases that might be treated by proton. What can you tell me?"

Joe gave him a quick synopsis.

"Of course while I was investigating treatments and particularly proton for my own case, my focus was on prostate cancer. But in the course of my research, and from my experience in Korea watching what was going on around me, I found out that there are several types of cancer that can be treated with proton beam therapy. Keep in mind that the peculiar characteristics of proton, as opposed to x-ray, or photon, radiation are the ability to focus the beam with fair precision, and the ability (because of the Bragg peak) to dictate the depth at which the proton beam will deliver its energy. These characteristics combine to greatly minimize damage to nearby healthy tissue, which means that the therapy can be used in close proximity to sensitive organs. In addition, while the research is still underway, it appears that doses can be increased because there is less danger to the surrounding tissue.

"Because of these characteristics, proton can be used for tumors that are close to vital organs, as would be the case with lung cancers that are near the heart, brain tumors, cancers of the neck or back that are near the spine, pancreatic cancer, chest and abdomen cancers, cancers of the eye, and so forth. And only recently, the Food and Drug Administration in the United States, which is responsible for approving medical treatments, approved the use of proton beam therapy for breast cancer. The characteristics of protons also give proton beam therapy a significant role in treating pediatric cases."

Joe proceeded to review the information he had relayed to the Garzas.

"I found a paper prepared by a doctor at the University of Pennsylvania outlining research on the side effects of proton therapy relative to other therapies - principally surgery and x-ray radiation - for a variety of cancers. As a rule, proton beam therapy either had no negative effect, or the incidence of negative side effects was considerably lower than it was for the alternatives.

"When I was in Korea," Joe concluded, "I saw a number of instances of cancers being treated with protons. Obviously some were prostate cases like my own, but there were other ones as well. Interestingly, some prostate cases were what they refer to as salvage proton cases. These were cases where the men had undergone surgery, but the surgery did not remove all the cancer. Because the body couldn't stand additional treatments, and because protons have fewer and less severe side effects, proton was being used to combat the remaining cancer. I also met a man who had a brain tumor that had not been treated for a number of years. When he arrived in Korea, he was unable to walk. But mid-way through his treatment, he was beginning to regain the use of his legs and was showing amazing progress.

"I also met a man who had a tumor at the base of his spine. It could not be removed surgically because of the location. With proton beam therapy, however, it was treated successfully."

They talked a little more, and then it was time to go. Bill asked Joe to keep him advised on the Garza boy's case, and Joe said he certainly would.

Joe returned to his office and found that there were no pressing issues. Before he left for home he called Mr. Garza, who told him that he had contacted both Dr. Siva and the oncologist and that they were sending the needed records to Mr. Poling to be forwarded to the National Cancer Center in Korea.

"I want to thank you for your assistance," said Mr. Garza, "and apologize to you for acting skeptical last night. As you can expect, since this whole incident began we have received all kinds of advice from our friends, as well as strangers. Some of it had to do with changes to diet and even voodoo magic. We had become somewhat careful about talking about the subject, but we felt it was necessary to explore every plausible sounding idea."

Joe agreed. "I, too, had to listen to a number of things, but I was able to focus on my own research to find a solution. Fortunately, I don't think I have lost any real friends over as a result of the process."

They ended the conversation by agreeing to keep each other informed.

On Wednesday of the following week, Joe heard from Mr. Garza.

"I have good news," he said. "I just received an email from Mr. Poling. He said that the medical team in Seoul has reviewed the medical information we sent last week and it appears that our son can be accepted for treatment. I also received an estimate of the cost which is about 40 or 50 percent of the cost I was expecting, based on what I had found out about the treatment centers in the United States. I worked it out with my father, and what we have raised so far will pay the cost. I won't need to pursue the tennis exhibition tournament."

"That certainly is great news," replied Joe. "When are you going to be able to go?"

"Well, there is a logistical issue. Normally this particular kind of cancer is treated with surgery, then chemotherapy, then radiation. Also, normally the proton center sees the patient for a consultation prior to starting treatment. This is when the diffuser and molds are made. Because we have not seen the doctors at the NCC yet, we will need to combine the consultation with the treatment phase.

"We have airline reservations for two weeks from tomorrow. We will all three travel to Korea and spend Christmas and New Year's there, and then I will have to come back in order to work. The consultation phase and the treatment phase will altogether take about six to eight weeks. As it nears the end of that period, I will travel again to Korea to bring the family home. I am very excited about the trip and the prospects for resolving my son's cancer.

"One thing I have learned, by the way, is that the plan in Korea now includes an English-speaking driver to take you back and forth from the apartment to the National Cancer Center. You still have to pay for the driver, but you won't have to go to the effort to find a reliable one with whom you can communicate. This will greatly help my wife, who may not adjust to the public transportation system as readily as you apparently did.

"We would like to invite you and your wife over for dinner tomorrow evening. And I hope that it will not be an imposition, but we will have many practical questions for you about traveling and staying in Korea."

"No problem at all," replied Joe. "Any time you need something, just let me know. I still have a file with all the brochures and information I used while I was there. I'll be happy to have you use them."

After they spoke, Joe called Maria to pass on the good news and the dinner invitation.

"That's wonderful," said Maria. "I'm going to call Rosario right away. Will you call Bill?"

"Yes. And I'll also stop on the way home for a couple more bottles of wine to take with us."

Joe called Bill and told him the good news, then went home, stopping to get the wine. When he got home, Maria had gone on an errand, so Joe went into the home office and started rummaging through his collection of maps and guidebooks from Korea so he would be ready to go see the Garzas the next evening.

Websites and resources Joe used to research pediatric cancer

Note: for updated information on websites and other information in this book, please see www.RoadToNamiIsland.blogspot.com.

Pediatric Proton Foundation - This organization promotes the use of proton beam therapy in combating pediatric (childhood) cancers - http://pediatricprotonfoundation.org/

National Association for Proton Therapy (NAPT) - www.proton-therapy.org/

General information on radiation therapy for childhood tumors - http://www.irsa.org/childhood_tumors.html

Natalie's Story - http://www.nataliescircleoflove.org/follow-natalies-journey/

Article: "Reduced Normal Tissue Toxicity With Proton Therapy" by James Metz, MD, The Abramson Cancer Center of the University of Pennsylvania - Posting Date: April 28, 2002; Last Modified: June 29, 2006 - http://protoninfo.com/Articles/UniversityofPennsylvania.pdf

CHAPTER 9. LESSONS LEARNED

It was New Year's Day. Joe had connected his laptop to the television set and was watching traditional New Year's Day programming from the United States. The girls and Maria had joined him to watch the Tournament of Roses Parade but left when the football games started. From time to time they wandered in to check on progress, they stayed only to watch the halftime shows.

The games themselves weren't particularly exciting, so Joe flipped from one to another to find the best ones and to keep up with what was going on. This New Year's Day was relatively peaceful. As he sat watching the television, Joe had the opportunity to reflect on the past year and to imagine what the coming year would bring.

Activity at work had picked up since he returned from Korea. His developer client had brought him one project immediately after his return and was now discussing another project with him. He had also just received notice that he was being included on a team of engineers and other specialists to investigate a bridge failure for the local highway department.

The girls were on their summer break and would be returning to school in March. They had completed the school year with very good grades and were already excited about the coming year. Victoria had taken a volunteer position for the summer in a veterinarian's office near their apartment. She loved animals and this was an opportunity to see if she might be interested in veterinary medicine as a career. Teresa had volunteered to help the school's tennis coach give lessons and was practicing whenever there was a spare moment. Maria was working at the school library during the summer but on an abbreviated schedule.

Joe and Maria had discussed again the idea of moving to the United States for college and had decided that now would be the time to make a visit to investigate the options. In the past, they had traveled to visit friends or see the sights, but they were now discussing a trip that would be more focused on schools. The plan that was developing in their conversations was to make a trip in February before the start of the school year. Schools in the United States would be in session, so it would be easier to see what campus activity was really like. On the other hand, they would need to watch the weather. This would be in the middle of winter in the United States and several of the schools they had discussed might be affected. They started talking up the plan with the girls, including discussion of what schools they might like to visit. The girls were thrilled.

Joe had discovered that he missed his experience in Korea. He had met some very nice people at the National Cancer Center and he had visited many interesting places. Joe sent several Christmas cards to staff members at the NCC, although he was not sure whether they were very familiar with the practice. He had gotten a letter or two after that and the technicians sent him a group photo of themselves.

Joe had gotten the idea of visiting Korea again, this time with Maria and the girls. He had not approached Maria about the idea yet, particularly because he had not figured out the logistics. Winter in Korea was pretty cold, but that was when the girls were out of school. Spring or Fall would be the best times to visit, but the girls were in school.

He reflected on his experiences with prostate cancer, including all the high and low moods. At mid-year he had been only vaguely aware of what a prostate gland was. By now, however, he knew pretty much everything a layman could possibly know about the prostate gland, the diseases of the prostate, prostate cancer, and the treatments, outcomes, and side effects of the various treatments.

His low moods included, of course, the day he learned that he in fact did have prostate cancer. This was a low point for a period of almost two months, starting when his family doctor told him there might be something wrong and extending until he was accepted for treatment at the National Cancer Center in Korea and had all the details straightened out. At least by then he had hope that his cancer would be addressed effectively. He had never really discussed it with Maria, but he remembered waking up in the middle of the night and lying in bed for hours worrying. He knew Maria loved him and supported him, but he was the one who was facing the disease and would be the one to die if the disease wasn't controlled.

He suddenly thought about Maria. She was a stalwart supporter, but he realized that she was probably helping him by stifling her own feelings so that he wouldn't worry more. He recalled that she was really excited when he got the news that he was going to Korea, and again when she took him to the airport to depart. It occurred to him just now that she was probably as relieved for herself and the girls as much as she was relieved for him. Joe realized that anything that made Maria truly happy made him happy too. What a lady. He decided to do something special for her. He smiled to himself.

Another low mood came from the saga of Bill's friend, Dennis. Joe saw some parallels between Dennis' story and his own at the beginning, but they quickly diverged. Dennis initially found out about his prostate problem in much the same way as had Joe. But Dennis received different advice and waited considerably longer to confirm and then deal with his cancer. Joe, on the other hand, pursued his research immediately and proactively and got answers. Joe wondered if he would have been less proactive if he had been advised to wait and monitor the disease. He was glad he hadn't.

The episode with Dennis had been especially distressing for Bill. Bill had two good friends going through prostate cancer challenges during the same span of time, although their outcomes were very different. While Bill would be happy that Joe had come out of the ordeal with a positive result, he was deeply saddened by Dennis' death.

To balance his low moods during the past six months, Joe had memories of some highs. The biggest ones were learning he was all set to go to Korea for his proton beam treatment, actually going, and best of all returning to Maria and the girls with his cancer under control. He reminded himself not to characterize his cancer as being "cured." He had been told many times that you don't cure cancer, because there might be microscopic stem cells that could begin to multiply and the cancer might return. He knew that he needed to get regular PSA tests to monitor this possibility. He was also comfortable that he knew how to research questions he might have and knew sources of information upon which he could rely.

One of the highest highs had occurred only recently when the Garzas left with their son for Korea. Joe and Maria had gone with several other friends to see them off at the airport just before Christmas. They were there now. Joe had gotten confirmation of their arrival and settling into the residential facility where they were staying, but he had not yet received any reports of progress in the treatment. Joe and Bill were to meet Mr. Garza at the airport in a few days when he returned. Joe was anxious to get a full report on how things were going but realized that it was still too early to get a medical report.

All these ideas were going around in his mind. In addition to the idea of visiting Korea again with the family, and the prospect of visiting campuses in the United States, Joe had been thinking about things he could do to use his newfound knowledge to help others. Even if he only helped one man seek screening and prevent a case of prostate cancer from going too far, he felt he would have achieved something important. But he hadn't figured out what he could do.

The phone rang. Joe started to get it, but before he could it stopped.

"It's Bill for you," said Maria from the doorway. "And after you're finished talking to him, can you come help me in the kitchen?"

"Of course," replied Joe as he got up and reached for the extension.

"Hello, Bill."

"Hey, Joe," said Bill. They still joked about this reference to the popular song from their college days. "I was just looking at my calendar and realized I'm in charge of programs at Rotary for the month of January. Can you put on a program for me? Normally, we eat and deal with one or two announcements and items of business, and then we have the program. The program should last only about twenty minutes, with questions, if that fits in. Most of the clubs in our area meet at nine PM, but fortunately our club meets at seven, so we should be through by nine."

Joe had visited some Rotary clubs over the years, usually with clients or other engineers.

"Yeah, I'm familiar with how they work, but what would you want me to talk about?" he asked.

"Why, prostate cancer, of course. Tell your story. It's going to be very useful and will be very much appreciated."

A light went on in Joe's head. This might be part of how he could use his knowledge to benefit others.

"Of course, I'll be happy to." Joe told Bill that he had been thinking about a way to help others get information on prostate cancer and the available remedies and added that this would be an excellent opportunity to do so.

"You know that I am comfortable making presentations in my business. I could prepare a PowerPoint presentation just like I would use for a client." They discussed a date that would be convenient for Joe during the coming month and some of the arrangements that would need to be made.

"The room we use for our weekly meetings is one of the function rooms at the hotel," said Bill, "and they have screens and other equipment, but you will probably need to use your own digital projector. I have seen people having problems with the hotel equipment from time to time. On the other hand, the audio equipment usually works fine."

They agreed to get together on the weekend to go over the presentation and to make more detailed plans.

After they hung up, Joe went into the kitchen to tell Maria about the conversation.

But first he asked, "How can I help?"

"I need you to pull out the ingredients to make your Mom's cornbread. You do remember what day it is, don't you, darling?"

"Of course," he said with relish. Joe's mother was born and raised in the southern United States, Alabama to be exact, and had strictly adhered to the southern tradition of ensuring luck for the New Year by dining on certain things on New Year's Day. Joe had brought this tradition into their marriage, and Maria thought it was just fine. Their version of the traditional menu included pork, greens, black-eyed peas, and fresh, hot cornbread made with the secret family recipe Joe had learned from his mother.

As he busied himself with his task, he told Maria about his conversation with Bill and the idea that had occurred to him.

"I've been looking for a constructive way I can make use of my experience with prostate cancer and help others," he said. "I have experience with speaking to groups and I know my way around PowerPoint presentations. I can give talks, particularly to men's groups, and encourage men to get PSA screenings and to act on the information they get. I can also encourage men to become more aware of their medical conditions and discuss them with their doctors so they make intelligent decisions about their treatment."

Maria had been listening intently. "You need to give those talks to men and women. I think that wives and girlfriends need to be aware of the choices that men face - actually that the family faces. When a man has prostate cancer, the rest of the family is affected."

"You're absolutely right. Marriage is a partnership; any relationship is a partnership. I should have thought of it that way," Joe replied.

"By the way, since you're going to make presentations, I forgot to tell you that I'm in charge of finding a program for the February meeting of the parent association at our school. March will be the back-to-school meeting, but February is not covered. I'm calling the program chairman right now and signing you up."

Joe agreed, but before he could say anything, the phone rang and he answered it. It was Bill.

"I just talked to my Rotary Club president. He was excited about the program lineup I have for January, but he wants your presentation to be as early as we can make it, perhaps next week. It will be the first meeting of the year. Are you game?"

Joe agreed and went to the home office to put both presentations in his calendar. When he returned, he stood in the middle of the kitchen and reviewed to himself what he would need to do to prepare the presentation. Joe was increasingly becoming excited by the prospect and almost missed the fact that the kitchen timer had sounded.

He pulled the cornbread out and tested it with a knife, pronouncing it ready. Maria and the girls were ready and the rest of the meal was already on the table. The objective was to serve the meal just when the hot cornbread was coming out of the oven.

They toasted the New Year with wine and ginger ale and proceeded to eat.

After they ate, Joe checked the status of the football games that were on and decided that they weren't important enough so he went into the office and gathered the information he would need to work on the presentation for Rotary.

During the week, Joe worked on the project and by Friday afternoon had gotten it into a condition that made him happy. He called Bill and they arranged to get together Saturday morning to review the results.

On the day of the Rotary meeting, Joe and Bill arrived early at the meeting location, which was the ballroom of one of the older hotels in Buenos Aires. The club was not the oldest one in the city, but it had been in existence for many years, and had a large membership of well-established business professionals.

Joe knew from long experience that it was a good idea to set up his equipment and practice his presentation several times before it came time to actually deliver the real thing. He did this with help from Bill to make sure the PowerPoint show could be easily seen and could be smoothly delivered once the room was full.

Just as he was finishing and putting his computer on standby, the first Rotarians started coming in the door. Soon the room was fairly full and the club members were mingling and discussing their Christmas and New Year's activities. A few came up to Bill and Joe and introduced themselves.

At the appointed time, the sergeant-at-arms rang the bell and announced that it was time for the meeting. Everyone took his or her seat and dinner was served.

Bill and Joe were seated at the head table with the club president and some other officers. Over dinner, Joe chatted with the president. He had met the gentleman before but only briefly. The dinner was followed by announcements and then the president asked Bill to introduce the program. Bill introduced Joe and explained that the program involved a subject he felt was vital for all the members of the club to know about.

Joe proceeded to make the presentation. "Thank you very much, Bill, for the introduction and thank you all in the club for having me as a speaker. I'm going to talk about a subject that is very, very important to you and is a matter of life and death.

"Let me summarize my story. Six months ago I knew very little about the prostate and prostate cancer. At that point, I received an indication that I might have something wrong with my prostate. Five months ago I received a confirmed diagnosis of prostate cancer. I then went through a process of deciding what to do. Four months ago I left on a journey to the National Cancer Center in Seoul, Korea, to be treated and was there for about two months. Since I returned home, I have been in good physical condition. My cancer is not cured in the common sense of the word, since cancer is never cured, however it is in remission. I will continue to monitor my cancer for the rest of my life, and with the Lord's help I will not have to go through any more experiences of this kind.

"I did a little bit of research on this club before I came to speak. I understand that there are about 150 members in the club, and counting just now there appear to be about that many here this evening. The statistics I am about to give do not apply to the few ladies that I see, but for the ladies, they apply to male family members: fathers, husbands, brothers, sons, and nephews, as well as male friends. So listen carefully.

"Looking around the room, I would guess that about half of the men here are younger than fifty, mostly thirties and forties, with a few younger men. The rest of you appear to be over fifties, mostly in your fifties and sixties with a few in your seventies. I'll use those numbers. In other words, half are younger than fifty and half are older than fifty.

"Statistically, according to a crude estimate based on the age distribution of this particular group and because you are older than the general population, about fifty of you (or about thirty-three percent) now have prostate cancer. Some of you know it and may have received or are receiving treatment. Some of you have it and don't know it. Another number of you do not have prostate cancer now but may get it in the future. I have seen a statistic that fifty percent of men over fifty and eighty percent of men over eighty have prostate cancer. Overall in the male population you can expect one in six will get it.

"Prostate cancer is the second leading type of cancer found in men, only after skin cancer, and it is the second leading cause of cancer deaths among men, second only to lung cancer. In addition, using statistics from the United States for a recent year, there are slightly more new cases of prostate cancer among men as there are new cases of breast cancer among women, both a little over two hundred thousand per year. And the death rates are similar: about fifteen percent for men with prostate cancer and nineteen percent for women with breast cancer.

"Let me address a couple of myths about prostate cancer. First, it is commonly thought of as an old man's disease. While it is true that the likelihood of contracting prostate cancer increases with age, it can affect younger men as well. This is important. Older men may get cancer but may die of other causes before they die of the cancer. Conversely, younger men with prostate cancer are more likely to die of the cancer if not treated effectively and quickly. Another myth is that it is a slow-growing disease and can be monitored rather than being actively addressed. While the disease is slower growing in about two-thirds of cases, it is more aggressive in a third of cases. In these cases delay of even a month or two may significantly and adversely impact the potential success of any treatment that is selected.

"What causes prostate cancer? No one has a definitive answer and there are no clear indicators, such as the link between smoking and cancers of the lungs, mouth, and throat. There are indications, still being researched, that there is a genetic link. If a male member of your family, such as your father or a brother, has had the disease, there is a higher probability that you will get it, and there is a higher probability that your sons will get it. There have also been some links suggested between lifestyle issues, such as diet, but these are still being studied and the possible relationships are not completely clear.

"For those of you who have received or are receiving treatment, you may have a pretty good idea of what is involved and what kinds of treatments are available. You may also be aware of the side effects of those forms of treatment. For those of you who have not been detected with cancer or who are yet to contract it, you probably know very little about it. This is not the principal topic of conversation between most men when they meet, and most men don't normally check books on this subject out of the library.

"How do you know that you have prostate cancer? What are the symptoms? Actually, you may have some of the symptoms, but they are subtle and you may not yet notice them. The urethra, the duct going from the bladder to the penis, goes directly through the prostate, so many symptoms are associated with urinary dysfunction. These may include the frequent need to urinate including needing to get up several times in the night to urinate; painful urination; difficulty in maintaining a stream; and difficulty in emptying the bladder. Other symptoms include a change in your ability to attain an erection and have the kind of sex you used to have.

"Also, some of the symptoms may be caused by other factors. For example, the frequent need to urinate may result from a bladder condition, a prostate problem other than cancer, or even diabetes. You may have one of these conditions and may have not yet determined that it is the cause.

"Fortunately, there are some simple screening tests to identify potential problems, and some more elaborate tests that can be used to provide early diagnoses and help determine the appropriate course of treatment. The most basic of these is the PSA test. I won't confuse you with the letters, but essentially this test can detect antigens produced by the prostate gland. If the number is high or increases dramatically, it is an indication of a problem that could be caused by a cancer. It can also be caused by other factors, including other prostate problems or even having sex too close to the time of taking the test. This test is a simple part of a routine blood test. You should ask that it be done on a regular basis when you have a blood test and certainly in connection with your regular annual physical exam.

"If the number is higher than normal or higher than normal for you as an individual or increases between tests your doctor should start investigating the reason. If your doctor doesn't investigate you should insist or find another doctor.

"Another common test is one most you are familiar with. Even if you are younger, you might have had a digital rectal exam, politely referred to as a DRE, when you joined the army. In this test, the doctor can feel the prostate which is adjacent to the rectum and is looking for abnormal hardness or roughness. I know we all dislike it when the doctor pulls out the rubber glove during our annual physical exam and asks us to bend over, but the information he gets from doing this could literally be the difference between living and dying. Take it like a man.

"If these tests raise suspicion, there are other tests that can be performed, including bone density tests, MRI and CT scans, and finally the biopsy. In the biopsy, several cores or samples are taken from the prostate and examined for evidence of cancer. If cancer is found, other information about the extent of the cancer can be determined.

"To recap: prostate cancer is a serious issue. It can be detected by being diligent, and if untreated or treated too late, it can kill you.

"Let me move then to the topic of what kinds of treatments are available for prostate cancer.

"The two most common treatments are surgery and radiation therapy. There are some other therapies that are used, but they are not always indicated for situations involving early detection and early action, which is the most desirable scenario. These other therapies include chemotherapy, hormone therapy, and biological therapy. The last one uses diet as a means of controlling the cancer, but it is still experimental. One traditional approach is called watchful waiting. This approach is more appropriate in situations where the man is older and is less likely to suffer from a slow-growing cancer than he is to die for another reason.

"Surgery is the most simple. I did some research and found that the first operation to remove a cancer-diseased prostate was performed in Tucson, Arizona, in 1893 by Dr. George Goodfellow. Surgery as a treatment for prostate cancer has become more sophisticated but has not materially changed since the time it was first practiced. Surgery usually involves removing the prostate gland and may involve removal of nearby tissue if there is an indication that it is diseased. The prostate is located in a delicate place, near other organs that are important, including the male reproductive system. Surgery is very delicate and difficult and can involve damage to nerves which control erections, bladder control, and the like. According to a study at the University of Pennsylvania, over 30 percent of men who undergo surgery lose their ability to control their bladders and about 60 percent become impotent.

"Turning to radiation; generally, radiation is used to ionize or damage the cancer cells. Unlike normal cells, cancer cells find it more difficult to reproduce when they have been damaged through ionization. While normal cells are more capable of overcoming damage and reproducing, radiation can damage them too. The strategy, then, is to deliver the radiation only to the cancer cells and avoid the normal cells. Various techniques have been developed to help achieve this.

"One technique is called brachytherapy, which involves inserting a number of tiny radioactive pellets or needles into the cancer itself. The radioactive needles then irradiate and ionize the cancer cells, thus killing the cancer. After a period of time, the needles lose their radioactivity and can be removed or simply left in position. The side effects include radioactivity being received by normal healthy cells in the vicinity. This can cause some of the same results as for surgery; namely damage to nerves and other tissues which are important to the male reproductive and urinary systems.

"Another radiation technique is use of an external x-ray beam to bombard the cancer and ionize the cancer cells. The problem here is to focus and direct the radiation sufficiently to affect the cancer cells without affecting the nearby normal tissue. Technology and improved computer control systems have made this process more precise.

"One of the problems with x-ray radiation is that the x-ray beam must travel through a certain amount of normal tissue before it reaches the target and then proceeds on through the body. This can cause radiation damage to healthy tissue cells on the way in and then on the way out. This undesired radiation can cause secondary cancers, as well as damage to healthy organs. Part of the solution to overcome this condition is to reduce the strength of the x-ray beam so that it will have a reduced effect on the healthy tissue. By doing this, however, the beam has less of an effect on the cancer.

"One more modern solution is to focus the beam and rapidly shoot it from different angles so that areas other than the tumor only receive a partial dose while the tumor receives a maximum dose. But the healthy tissue still receives some radiation and the side effects remain, even though to a lesser extent.

"As a result of World War II, new knowledge in atomic science led Robert R. Wilson, a physicist involved in the Manhattan Project, to suggest in 1947 that proton beams could have value in medical applications. The proton beam is created by stripping protons from hydrogen atoms and accelerating and releasing them as a beam. Unlike an x-ray beam, which is a beam of energy, the proton beam is a beam of charged particles that deliver energy at a certain point.

"The proton beam has an interesting characteristic. The beam delivers very little energy until it reaches a point known as the 'Bragg peak.' When it reaches that point, it delivers all of its energy in a very short distance and then is finished. By controlling the point at which the Bragg peak occurs, the beam can be made to deliver its energy to the cancer cells and greatly minimize the impact on surrounding normal cells. In addition to controlling the depth at which the beam delivers its energy, the beam can be passed through a diffuser to make its shape conform to the shape of the target cancer. Because the energy is delivered almost exclusively to the desired target, a much greater amount of energy can be delivered in each dose.

"Incidentally, as an exciting improvement on this technique, advances in computer technology will soon allow the computer to adjust the shape of the beam as well as the depth for its target. This new technology is called IMPT (for intensely modulated proton therapy) and is especially beneficial for complex tumor shapes, such as head-and-neck tumors, tumors of the lower abdomen that have a curved shape, and tumors wrapped around the spinal cord or brain stem. IMPT can shape complex fields with a limited number of radiation angles, which keeps the treatment time as short as possible and helps to spare healthy tissue. This technology gives clinicians more options for delivering the dose more precisely in order to spare more healthy tissue in the course of delivering treatments.

"Various experiments and efforts were made in the 1960s and 1970s to use proton beam technology for medical purposes, but it wasn't until the last decade of the 20th century that a functional hospital-based proton center was developed at the Loma Linda University Medical Center in California, United States. Since the turn of the new century, several additional centers became operational, and to date there are nine such centers in the United States, one in Germany, and one in Korea. Several others are under development, and the number will rise over the next few years.

"Proton beam therapy is an ideal method for addressing a number of kinds of cancer. Generally, it is most desirable for cancers that are located deeper in the body at a fixed point or that are close to a vital organ, such as the heart or the brain. It does not work with cancers that by their nature are spread throughout the body, such as cancers of the blood, or that have metastasized or spread out from the original location. Finally, proton beam therapy is ideal for pediatric cancers because the ability to control the beam is vital in avoiding adverse effects on the still-developing organs in young children. In fact, we are acquainted with a local family whose young son is right now in Korea getting treated for a brain tumor. He is a little over half way through his treatment and the reports are that it appears to be shrinking.

"I chose to have my prostate cancer treated by proton beam therapy because the side effects are extremely limited. Statistically, only half as many men are affected by impotence as is the case with either external beam radiation or surgery, and less than one percent suffer from incontinence, or the ability to control the bladder.

"I also chose to go to Korea for treatment. To make this decision, I considered a number of criteria that were important to me, including:

Accessibility - how easy it is to get to a center. I note that none are currently available in South America.

Delay - how long one has to wait to get treatment

Qualifications - of center personnel

Advancements in Treatment - does the center keep up with and use information about advances in therapy

Cost

Intangible Element - other factors concerning overall livability of the center's community and the quality of the experience, particularly when your situation does not allow you to live at home and receive treatment on an outpatient basis.

"I was very happy with my treatment experience. I suffered no observable side effects of the proton beam therapy. Various tests have shown that there is no evidence at this point of any remaining cancer. I will be taking my first post-treatment PSA test in about a month, three months after concluding my treatment. I will monitor my PSA level for the rest of my life.

"Let me briefly describe my experience at the National Cancer Center in Seoul. I arrived in Korea and was met by one of the members of the concierge staff of the Center and taken to my apartment. One of the advantages of treatment in Korea is that your accommodations for the eight weeks you are there are included in the price of treatment. Also, your trips between the apartment and the proton beam therapy center at the National Cancer Center are included. This means that you are only responsible for your food, entertainment, and travel. This greatly reduces your cost of being treated and reduces the risk of surprises regarding costs.

"The apartment was fully furnished and included various services, such as cleaning. The building had a gym/exercise center with exercise equipment, squash courts, indoor tennis, and a pool. The apartment also provides a business center that facilitates your work activities. Finally, it is located close to stores, restaurants, and other services. The apartment provided shuttle service to many locations, including shopping. My travel within Seoul and throughout Korea was easy because of the extensive public transportation system. My treatment was quick and orderly. I was able to spend my afternoons and weekends seeing the sights and enjoying the culture of Korea.

"I was very much impressed with Korea as a travel destination and plan to go back. The people are friendly and polite and extremely helpful. While I was there I visited the Demilitarized Zone (or DMZ) that separates North and South Korea; Pyeongchang, the site of the 2018 Winter Olympics; the port city of Busan; as well as many interesting places within Seoul. I visited many of the museums, shopping districts, and restaurants, and I had many opportunities to observe Korean culture. I felt that, although my travel to Korea was primarily for the purpose of receiving treatment, it was a valuable educational experience.

"I'm going to run a slide show on the screen of photographs of the many places I went and the things that I did, but I'm not going to narrate it. While the show is running I'll take questions. Bill and I will both stay here after the meeting in case anyone has additional questions.

"So to close, let me reiterate some points: First, all men, especially once they reach the age of 50 should seek to be screened regularly with PSA tests. Second, if there is any indication of a problem, either by a high PSA count or by a count that is increasing, make your doctor investigate the cause. Third, be aware of your health conditions and make wise decisions generally. Fourth, if you discover that you have prostate cancer and qualify for proton beam treatment, consider that it has been shown to be effective and has fewer side effects than other forms of treatment. And finally, fifth, if you select proton beam therapy, consider the advantages of seeking treatment at the National Cancer Center in Seoul, Korea."

"Are there any questions?"

No one had any questions that they wanted to ask from the floor, so the club president officially adjourned the meeting. Several people from the audience then gathered around Joe and Bill to talk and ask questions. The club president joined the group.

"That was very informative. Have you considered writing a book?" asked the president. Joe had not even thought of it until the question was raised.

"Well no, I hadn't, but I have decided to do whatever I can to get the word out to men, particularly on the need for screening and early action. Writing a book might be a way to accomplish that."

A lady from the audience came up and said her husband was having some problems and had wished he could attend, but he wasn't able to come this evening, so he had asked her to attend and take notes. She asked if she could get a copy of the PowerPoint presentation. Joe said he could email a copy to her and would also send her a copy of his speech.

Three men came up to ask about the symptoms Joe had described. They talked, and Joe advised them all to see their doctors and have a PSA test done as soon as possible. If any problems were indicated from this type of screening, they would be referred to a urologist for further investigation. He reminded them that they should be persistent until they got answers to any questions they had.

After they left, a man who had been standing on the edge of the group approached Joe.

"I was recently diagnosed with prostate cancer and I have been researching my options, just as you did," he explained. "My concern is that I have been reading about how proton treatments are delivered at the various facilities, and I am becoming confused by the differences. As an example, I don't understand why some facilities use gold markers to guide the beam and other facilities use other methods. Also, some use an inflatable device to stabilize the prostate and others use another system. How can I understand which procedures are better and what is appropriate for me?"

Joe surveyed the man and then slowly responded. "I have come across these kinds of questions in various blogs as I did my research. You need to step back and look at the bigger picture. Each facility has some differences in its practices and procedures, but these details are not as important as the bigger issue. You have been presented with a method for resolving your disease. It may be the best method available to you. Certainly, it is the method with the lowest incidence of side effects. If you qualify for it, you need to find a way to move forward expeditiously to get the treatment. It could potentially save your life, and saving your life is more important than the details. I wish you the best of luck, my friend."

When the man left, Joe turned to Bill.

"It reminds me of a situation I dealt with in my engineering career. I was working with a committee that was trying to figure out where to locate a toll bridge, but the committee kept focusing on what type of bridge structure would be used. They couldn't understand that the design of the bridge would be influenced by the location, not the other way around. Our engineering team joked that they were caught up in determining what color uniform the toll taker would wear. Proton beam therapy is proton beam therapy. If it is best for you, pursue it."

After the room had cleared, Joe and Bill packed the equipment and hauled it to Joe's car.

"Let me treat you to a cup of coffee," said Bill. "You put on an excellent presentation."

They went to the hotel coffee shop and ordered.

"I have to talk a little," said Joe when they had been served. "I keep thinking that prostate cancer is a death sentence. It may not kill you today or tomorrow, but it will get you eventually. If you hold out long enough, you might die of something else first, like being hit by a bus, but the prostate cancer is waiting there to get you eventually. If you don't do something about it quickly and decisively, your chances of prevailing diminish. Living with a cancerous prostate is not really living. You will have to be vigilant constantly to make sure it doesn't turn worse. If your cancer has metastasized, you may need chemotherapy and/or hormone therapy. When it turns worse you will be faced with pain and suffering as you die. Of course, you know all this now because of how closely you were involved with Dennis' experience.

"I keep thinking about how close I came to eventually ending up like Dennis. During the entire time I was dealing with the prostate cancer I didn't really feel sick or show any obvious symptoms. I was going to the bathroom more, but it was so gradual a change I didn't even think about it until the urologist asked me about it. It was lucky that I had a physical and that Doctor Silva had been routinely including a PSA test in the blood work. When all this started, I didn't even know what PSA was. If things had gone differently, I could have gone on a long time and when I finally learned I had it, it would have been too late.

"I firmly believe that the stuff I stressed in the presentation is right-on. First, men need to be screened regularly with PSA tests. Second, if a problem is indicated, whether a high PSA or a PSA that is increasing, men need to see a urologist. Third, men need to take charge of their decisions about health care and make sure they know all about the choices for treatment that are available to them. Fourth, if they get a diagnosis of prostate cancer, they need to determine if they qualify for proton beam therapy. If they qualify, they need to strongly consider that option. Fifth, if proton beam therapy is appropriate, they need to consider being treated at the National Cancer Center in Seoul."

Joe paused and sipped from his coffee.

"I guess, when you boil it down, it's a matter of awareness. Awareness of your PSA and awareness of your choices. If you know what your choices are, most people can make reasonable, intelligent decisions."

He paused again.

"Maybe I will write a book. If it helps one man it will be worth it."

Joe raised his cup. "To the memory of Dennis."

"To Dennis," responded Bill.

Websites with other information on proton beam therapy for cancer

Note: for updated information on websites and other information in this book, please see www.RoadToNamiIsland.blogspot.com.

http://affordableprotontherapy.blogspot.com/

http://dailycaller.com/2010/10/05/breast-cancer-receives-much-more-research-funding-publicity-than-prostate-cancer-despite-similar-number-of-victims/

http://www.prostate-cancer.org/education/localdis/brosman_RP2003.html

EPILOGUE

In late January Joe found out that the Garza's son was making good progress. Mrs. Garza and the boy had been in Korea since Christmas, while Mr. Garza had returned to Argentina to work. Joe and Maria had invited Mr. Garza over for dinner on several occasions. He told them that several families had done this, and that he was afraid he was gaining weight from all the good cooking. Joe had an ulterior motive in having Mr. Garza over as this was a way to get caught up on the boy's progress and to find out Mr. Garza's reaction to working with the staff at the NCC. In February, as the treatment process neared its end, Mr. Garza went back to Korea for a week and returned with his wife and son. A scan at the end of the proton treatment showed no visible tumor and the proton radiation oncologists expressed optimism for the boy's full recovery.

After the family returned, the Garza boy was scheduled to undergo six rounds of chemotherapy over a period of three months. His parents were looking forward to the completion of the chemotherapy and a determination that his case was NED, which stands for no evidence of disease. The Garzas knew that their son would be dealing with doctors over the rest of his life to monitor for possible side effects and for any possible relapse. They were happy, however, that the choice of proton therapy reduced the scope of side effects and that most would be attributable to the chemotherapy. Neurocognitive tests in the future would determine if there would be any effects on the boy's mental and physical growth.

In February three months had passed since Joe's own treatment, and he went to his urologist for his first tests. He would be taking these tests every three months for the rest of his life. Joe found that his PSA had dropped to 3.8, a 60 percent drop from what it had been prior to his treatment. He understood that he should continue to experience reductions at each test until about 18 to 24 months after treatment when he would reach his nadir, or lowest point for his PSA level. After that, it should remain stable but would continue to be monitored.

Buoyed by the results, Joe and Maria discussed with the girls the thought they had long held about moving to the United States before the girls reached college age. The consensus was that now was a good time. Accordingly, the girls did not start the regular school term in March, since they would be starting in September in America. To keep their studying skills honed, the girls each took on a project to pursue in the interim.

Teresa quickly suggested that she would like to study Korea as her project. She showed the others her laptop computer and the collection of photographs Joe had sent while he was there. She had organized the photos to correspond with the emails and explanations Joe had sent, along with her own notes of their Skype conversations. Teresa and her parents decided that she would collect information on Korea and make a PowerPoint presentation using information gathered in her research. Perhaps she could even write an article for a magazine aimed at secondary school students.

Victoria had some more difficulty in choosing a project and decided to continue volunteering at the veterinarian's office for the time being. Joe and Maria thought that this would be a good alternative, at least for now.

Joe proceeded to sell his business. He had met several engineers from a firm located in Rio de Janeiro while he was working on the site evaluation project for his developer client the previous year. They began a conversation at the time because the firm was interested in establishing an office in Buenos Aires and Joe knew he would eventually be interested in selling his business. The deal came together smoothly, which gratified Joe. He took on two engineers who relocated from Rio to Argentina, training them on the nuances of the business locally and introducing them to his clients and the projects that he had in the pipeline. It helped that his assistant developed a good relationship with the two new men and they appeared to work well together. As part of the deal, Joe agreed to remain under contract as a consultant to the firm for a period of five years on an on-call basis.

In April, Joe took Maria and the girls to Korea on vacation for three weeks. They visited many places in Seoul with which Joe was familiar, including many of the museums, the shopping areas at Itaewon, and the COEX Mall. They also visited the parks where the girls played a considerable amount of tennis. They went to the top of the North Seoul Tower and went sightseeing on the Seoul City Bus Tour. A few evenings were spent walking along the river observing the lights on the bridges.

They were in Korea during the Lotus Lantern Festival, honoring the birthday of Buddha. They observed demonstrations of lantern making, visited flea markets, and a Nori-Madang, or outdoor stage festival. They watched a procession of Buddhist monks carrying lanterns from Chogyesa Temple and along Chongno Street.

They also visited several sites associated with the Korean War and the Demilitarized Zone. Teresa was particularly happy as she was able to explain many of the sites and their significance from her research. She also appreciated the extensive exhibits at the Korean National Museum and insisted that they go back more than once.

Finally, they took a local ferry to Nami Island. Joe had wanted to do this while he was in Seoul undergoing treatment, but never got around to it. This was essentially a day trip, starting with a bus trip from Seoul and a short ferry ride to the Island.

Nami Island is an island in the Bukhangang River formed when the Cheonpyeong Dam was built. It is about ten miles (six kilometers) in circumference and has meadows and forests with several varieties of trees. A popular Korean TV series (Winter Love Song) was filmed there, increasing the popularity of the Island. Artifacts and locations used in the show are featured.

Nami Island was named after General Nami, whose grave is on the island. Nami was a young military leader who made a name for himself and died early during the Joseon Dynasty in the middle 15th century.

The visit to the island gave the family the opportunity to relax and enjoy a beautiful spring day while expanding their experience in Korean culture.

During their trip, Joe took them to the National Cancer Center and introduced them to some of the staff who had taken care of him during his treatment. Maria and the girls enjoyed seeing where Joe had been and meeting the staff. At the same time, the staff members were happy to have the opportunity to meet Joe's family, about whom he had spoken so much during his stay.

On the trip home to Argentina, Joe spoke to Maria about his feelings of returning to Seoul.

"It's funny, and I really wouldn't have expected it to happen this way, but I found that I really missed Korea and the people, particularly the people I knew at the National Cancer Center. I was talking to some of them when we were at the graduation party for the patients. They told me that some of the other patients had expressed interest in moving to Korea, or at least returning there with their families. I can see that. We will need to go again. I still want to get to Jeju Island."

"I can see why you loved it," replied Maria. "It's like they are your family in Korea. I'd like to go back again myself. I found it to be a very fascinating place."

When they returned to Buenos Aires, they set about making preparations for moving to the United States and proceeded to move in June. They initially moved in with Joe's father in Peoria, Illinois. He was getting elderly and they could help take care of him while they adjusted to their new home. Eventually, they decided, they would probably move into their own house or apartment, but for the time being his father's house was large enough and would do nicely for them all.

After they moved, Victoria took a noncredit course at the local community college in American history and government for background. She also took an online course in study strategies and habits to help her acclimate herself to the American school system. In the Fall she began her senior year in high school. Teresa started the Fall semester as a tenth grader but adjusted a number of classes to offset the difference in the levels of work; in some areas she was ahead of her classmates and in some areas she was behind. Both girls were intelligent and adjusted well to school and to their new schoolmates, especially when the tennis coach found out they were talented tennis players and could bolster the fortunes of the tennis team.

One thing Joe thought he would leave behind in Buenos Aires was his activities in support of prostate cancer awareness. He had been developing contacts with groups interested in men's health and cancer awareness and had expected these activities to fade away. To his surprise, however, he discovered when he moved that there was a growing need for such advocacy in the United States as well. True, while insurance programs in the United States typically would not pay for treatment at the National Cancer Center in Korea, there were many men who needed to learn about the availability of and benefits of proton beam treatment. Also, some men didn't have insurance that would pay for their treatment and cost considerations suggested that they consider treatment in Korea. More importantly, there needed to be a constant advocacy in support of the need for screening for early detection of cancer.

Joe also learned quickly that there was need for advocacy of proton beam treatments for other cancers, particularly pediatric cancer. Joe's experience with the Garza boy showed this, but he found it to be true as well in the United States. Even though there were many more proton beam facilities in America, pediatricians and pediatric oncologists were still inadequately aware of the benefits of this form of treatment. Joe quickly joined some local groups providing support to families with children with cancer and helped assist them and their doctors in making contact with appropriate experts. He also created and delivered presentations on pediatric cancers and proton therapy.

One evening in the early Fall Joe and Maria were sitting on the patio at Joe's father's house, having a glass of wine. The girls had settled into their school routine, and Joe and Maria were making a smooth transition to their new life.

"You realize, don't you," said Joe with a sigh of contentment, "that this is right about the time last year that I was starting treatment in Seoul. A lot of water has gone under the bridge since then."

"I am aware of that," said Maria.

"I don't know if I have said as strongly as I need to that I appreciate all the love and support you have given me during this ordeal. I think that the support from you and the girls has to be a part of the reason everything has gone as well as it has. I can't imagine going through this without you, and I don't want to imagine what it would be like for you if I hadn't gotten through it."

"Well, we're just glad you're here," said Maria.

"I think a lot about what has happened," he continued. "It's like I have been released from my burdens to follow a new path. Do you remember the movie *Castaway* we saw last year? Tom Hanks was some sort of low or mid-level executive for Federal Express. He caught a ride on one of their airplanes to go somewhere, but the airplane crashed in the ocean. He was the only survivor and found himself deserted on an island. He was able to salvage some of the goods from the airplane in order to survive, and he was stranded there for seven years. During that time, he had two things that gave him purpose and kept him going. One was to get back to his girlfriend and the other was to deliver one of the packages that was on the plane. When he was finally rescued, he went to see his girlfriend and found that she had married. Then he went and found the person to whom the package was addressed and delivered the package. At the end, after dealing with these two objectives, he was driving across an open area and stopped at an intersection in the middle of nowhere, got out of the car and stood in the middle of the intersection and yelled with his arms outstretched, signifying his release for his long-standing obligations and his opportunity for the future. That's the way I feel."

Maria squeezed his hand and smiled.

Websites

Note: for updated information on websites and other information in this book, please see www.RoadToNamiIsland.blogspot.com.

Itaewon Shopping District - http://visitkorea.or.kr/enu/SH/SH_EN_7_2_6_1.jsp

Seoul City Bus Tour - http://en.seoulcitybus.com/sub.php?PN=introduction_sctb&mainNum=1&subNum=11

Nami Island - http://www.lifeinkorea.com/Travel2/365

APPENDIX A - GLOSSARY OF TERMS

Caution: These are necessarily brief and elementary definitions, provided to assist readers of this book. For further information on any of these words or terms, consult medical and scientific sources or speak with your doctor. Note that the National Cancer Institute has an online dictionary of cancer terms at http://www.cancer.gov/dictionary.

Biologic Therapy - Treatment for disease (cancer) utilizing diet and supplements to reduce the tumor and/or limit its spread.

Biopsy - A procedure by which one or more cores or samples are removed from the prostate through the rectum to verify that that cancer is present and to determine the extent and progress of the cancer.

BPH (Benign Prostatic Hyperplasia) - A condition in which the prostate gland enlarges, creating interference with the urethra. Some of the symptoms of BPH are similar to those of prostate cancer.

Brachytherapy - A form of internal radiation in which radioactive needles or seeds are placed in the cancer. Over time, the radioactivity ionizes the cancer cells. Eventually, the radioactivity diminishes and the seeds may be left in place or removed.

Bragg Peak - A unique characteristic of the proton beam whereby the beam of particles delivers very little energy until it reaches a certain point at which almost all of its energy is delivered, after which point very little energy remains. The operator of the beam adjusts it so the Bragg peak coincides with the location of the targeted tumor. This allows a larger dose to be delivered since there is greatly reduced impact on healthy tissues that lie before or beyond the target cancer.

Chemotherapy - Treatment for disease (cancer) utilizing chemicals that kill cancer cells.

Cryosurgery (or Cryotherapy) - Treatment for disease (cancer) utilizing extreme cold to kill abnormal cells.

CT Scan (Computerized Tomography) - A technique using multiple X-ray images from different angles to produce an image of conditions in the body.

Cyberknife - A proprietary form of external radiation (X-ray) which is delivered through a series of bursts from different directions so that all the radiation is delivered to the tumor but the other areas of the body receive only a portion of the radiation. This reduces the amount of radiation delivered to individual areas of non-cancerous tissue, but increases the number of areas through which radiation will pass.

Digital Rectal Exam (DRE) - A test performed by a physician in which he inserts his finger in the patient's rectum to probe those parts of the prostate that can be reached. The physician is looking for any indication of irregular hardness or roughness that might indicate a cancer or other condition.

DMC Ville - The apartment facility in Korea used by the NCC to house foreign patients being treated.

DRE - see Digital Rectal Exam.

Drug Therapy - Treatment for disease (cancer) utilizing drugs.

Erectile Dysfunction - Failure of the man's penis to achieve a satisfactory erection. The erection is controlled by nerves and blood vessels in the vicinity of the prostate. These may be damaged through surgery or X-rays.

Gleason Score - A system for characterizing and quantifying the aggressiveness of a cancer case ascertained by the analysis of biopsy samples. In conducting the analysis, a score of 1 to 5 is given to the sample that is most involved with the disease and a second score is given to the second most involved sample. The two scores are added to produce a composite score of between 2 and 10, which is the Gleason score.

HIFU (High Intensity Focused Ultrasound) - Treatment for disease (cancer) utilizing a method for heating the tumor, thereby destroying cancerous cells.

Hormone Therapy - Treatment for disease (cancer) utilizing hormones to reduce the tumor and/or limit its spread.

Hospice - A facility for housing and caring for terminally ill patients as they near the end of their lives.

IMPT (Intensity Modulated Proton Therapy) - A new technique for aiming the proton beam during a treatment session, replacing the diffuser with a computer controlled method. The technique is faster and more accurate than the use of the physical diffuser to configure the beam's shape.

IMRT (Intensity Modulated Radiation Therapy) - A new technique for aiming a beam of X-rays to more precisely configure the beam to conform to the shape of the tumor.

Incontinence - A condition in which a person cannot control bladder and/or bowel functions and may need to wear adult diapers or use other protection. The urethra, bladder, and intestines are located close to the prostate and can be affected by surgery or X-rays.

KMI International - An organization operating under the direction of the government of South Korea and responsible for providing facilities and promoting use of Korean medical facilities by foreign patients. Mr. Curtis Poling is the KMI International representative in the United States and provides assistance to patients and potential patients seeking information on treatment in Korea.

KTO (Korea Tourism Organization) - An organization operating under the government of South Korea responsible for promotion of tourism in Korea.

Metastasis (variations: Metastatic, Metastases, Metastasized) - The condition of a cancer in which it has spread elsewhere in the body from the original tumor. Certain forms of treatment cannot be used if the cancer has metastasized.

MRI (Magnetic Resonance Imaging) - A technique using radio waves and computer analysis to develop an image of features inside the body. This technique is especially useful for imaging soft tissue, as opposed to X-rays which are better for imaging bones and hard features.

NAPT (National Association for Proton Therapy) - An organization providing information on proton beam therapy and about the facilities that deliver proton beam therapy to patients, usually cancer patients.

NCC (National Cancer Center) - A medical center located in Seoul, Korea, and one of eleven facilities worldwide offering proton beam therapy.

Oncologist - A doctor specializing in cancer and the treatment of cancer.

Pediatric Cancers - Cancers experienced by children. A particular difficulty in treating such cancers results from the fact that the child's body is still growing and developing and is more susceptible to the side effects of some cancer treatments.

Pediatric Proton Foundation - An organization providing information and assistance to families of children who might be able to be treated with proton beam therapy for pediatric cancers.

Photon - A bundle of electromagnetic energy. While a photon is not technically a particle, it can have the characteristics of particles, as when it collides with electrons or other particles. In cancer treatment, the photon beam (X-ray) ionizes the cancer cells leaving them unable to divide. Unable to grow, the cancer then withers away.

Prostate - A gland located generally between the bladder and the penis and surrounding the urethra.

Prostate Cancer - A cancer that can develop within the prostate gland, but may affect tissue immediately adjacent and can ultimately spread throughout the body (metastasize).

Prostate Specific Antigens - see PSA.

Prostatectomy - A surgical procedure in which all or a portion of the prostate is removed, sometimes accompanied by the removal of lymph nodes and/or other tissue in the vicinity which appears to be cancerous. Removal of the entire prostate is referred to as "radical prostatectomy."

Proton Beam Therapy (PBT) - Treatment for disease (cancer) utilizing a beam of protons to ionize cancer cells. Unlike x-ray (photon) radiation which is a beam of energy, the beam of protons does not deliver its energy evenly, but delivers it within a short distance at a point known as the "Bragg peak," thus having little effect on tissue through which it passes leading up to the target or beyond the target.

PSA; PSA Test - Measures Prostate Specific Antigens and is an indicator of possible prostate problems.

Radiation Therapy - Treatment for disease (cancer) utilizing radiation to ionize cancer cells. This prevents the cells from being able to divide and causes the tumor to wither away. Radiation therapy may be delivered from outside the body (external) as with X-rays, or from inside the body (internal) as with brachytherapy.

Sexual Dysfunction - Any condition in which sexual organs and processes fail to operate properly, as in erectile dysfunction.

Side Effects - Effects caused by various forms of treatment other than the desired effect of eliminating the disease. Some common side effects of cancer treatments are fatigue, pain, nausea, vomiting, decreased blood cell counts, hair loss, and mouth sores. Other side effects may include incontinence, impotence, and erectile dysfunction.

Soju - An alcoholic drink that is popular in Korea. Soju is made primarily from rice and tastes like vodka, but sweeter.

Staging - A method of characterizing the nature and extent of growth of a cancer to facilitate communication among medical professionals on the status of particular cases. While the system is similar for different types of cancers, the levels of quantification and the thresholds for different responses vary between cancers.

Surgery - Treatment for disease (cancer) involving the removal of diseased (cancerous) tissue, sometimes along with other nearby tissues that may be diseased. See Prostatectomy.

Urologist - A doctor specializing in the treatment of diseases affecting a man's urinary tract, including those affecting the prostate.

Watchful Waiting - A strategy for dealing with prostate cancer by not taking overt action. In some situations, a slow growing cancer will not cause severe adverse consequences during the remaining normal lifetime of the patient. If this is the case, it may be better to simply monitor the progress of the disease and slow its progress with hormone treatments. This approach avoids complications due to undesirable side effects of other forms of treatment. The expectation is that any change in the status of the disease can be identified and other treatment methods pursued before the disease becomes unmanageable.

APPENDIX B - PEOPLE INVOLVED IN PROTON BEAM THERAPY

1. Following is a list of organizations and real people involved in the growing use of proton beam therapy for treatment of cancers, including prostate cancer. Many of these appear in the book.

KMI - A private corporation which operates hospitals in South Korea and China, provides medical services, and assists in marketing medical tourism services.

Korean Tourism Organization (KTO) - A South Korean government organization promoting tourism in South Korea and providing a source of information for those planning to visit Korea for medical or other purposes.

National Cancer Center (NCC) - A South Korean government organization that operates hospitals and cancer treatment facilities throughout South Korea, operates research and treatment programs, and monitors cancer trends for the government.

Mr. Leonard Artz, Executive Director, National Association for Proton Therapy (NAPT), Silver Spring, Maryland, United States - Mr. Artz has extensive experience in understanding the science of protons and their application to proton beam therapy. The association he heads is an advocate for the development and application of this technology in treating a variety of diseases, primarily cancer.

Dr. Cho Kwan Ho (Dr. Cho), Radiation Oncologist, National Cancer Center, Seoul, South Korea - Dr. Cho treats patients with several types of cancers, including lung, head and neck, central nervous system, and prostate cancers. Before returning to Korea, Dr. Cho was a professor at the University of Minnesota for thirteen years. Dr. Cho is licensed to practice in Korea, as well as Minnesota and California in the United States. He is a member of the Korean Medical Association, the American Medical Association, and the Minnesota Medical Association, and is Board Certified by the Korean Board of Radiation Oncology, and by the American Board of Radiology in Radiation Oncology. Dr. Cho has additional memberships in the Korean Society of Head and Neck Oncology, the Korean Society of Therapeutic Radiation, the Korean Cancer Research Association, the American Society for Therapeutic

Radiology and Oncology, the International Society for Radiosurgery, and the Society for Neuro-oncology in the United States.

Mr. Han Man Jin (Mr. Han), Chairman of KMI International, South Korea - Mr. Han has been supporting patient care and overall patient services, arranging media support and other governmental support to ensure medical services in Korea meet a high standard.

Mr. Jin Soo Nam (Mr. Jin), Executive Director of the KTO - Mr. Jin has significant responsibility for developing Korea's medical tourism. He has directed Proton Beam Therapy Project with hospitals and global health care agencies.

Dr. Kim Dae Yong (Dr. Kim), Office of Planning and Coordination at the National Cancer Center, Seoul, South Korea - Dr. Kim is a member of the American Society of Therapeutic Radiology and Oncology and a past member of the European Society of Therapeutic Radiology and Oncology. Dr. Kim is also a member of the Korean Society of Therapeutic Radiology and Oncology, and serves or has served on the Examination Affairs Committee, the Information Affairs Committee, the Quality Assurance Committee, and the Scientific Affairs Committee. Dr. Kim served on the Scientific Affairs Committee of the Liver Cancer Study Group and serves on the Colorectal Cancer Committee of the Korean Cancer Study Group.

Dr. Kim Joo Young (Dr. Kim), Head of the Center for Proton Therapy at the National Cancer Center, Seoul, Korea - Dr. Kim is a member of the Korean Society of Radiation Oncology and the European Society of Radiation Oncology.

Lee Sang-Mi (Wendy) and Han Young-Wook (Young Wook) - The concierges working with patients at the National Cancer Center in Seoul, Korea.

Mr. Noh Kyong-Tae (Mr. Noh), Marketing Director, KMI International, Seoul, South Korea and St. Simons Island, Georgia, United States – Mr. Noah is in charge of non-medical patient services for the National Cancer Center (NCC), and supervises the concierges. Mr. Noah works with Mr. Curtis Poling to assist foreign patients of the NCC.

Mr. Park Hyun Chul (Mr. Park), CEO of KMI International, South Korea - Mr. Park is a professional consultant in Korean health care institutions and services. Based on his knowledge and experience, he has been a leading adviser to the proton beam therapy project and medical tourism industry.

Mr. Curtis Poling, CEO of KMI International, St. Simons Island, Georgia, United States - Mr. Poling is a prostate cancer survivor who was treated with proton beam therapy at the Loma Linda University Hospital in California, United States. After being treated, Mr. Poling became an advocate for proton beam therapy and has assisted several patients in traveling to Korea for treatment by the National Cancer Center in Seoul.

Mrs. Susan Ralston, Executive Director and Founder, Pediatric Proton Foundation, Virginia Beach, Virginia, United States - Mrs. Ralston became interested in proton beam therapy as a treatment for pediatric cancers and organized the Pediatric Proton Foundation to provide information and advocacy for pediatric patients and their families. Mrs. Ralston's interest began when her son contracted Ewing's Sarcoma. She researched the disease and potential treatments and discovered proton beam therapy. Mrs. Ralston serves on the Board of the Hampton University Proton Therapy Institute in Hampton, Virginia, United Sates.

2. Following is a list of the fictional characters in this book, through whom we are telling the story of proton beam therapy and its use in treating prostate cancer and other cancers.

Joe - American living in Argentina for last thirty years. Joe is a civil and mechanical engineer working as an independent consultant on development and construction projects throughout South America.

Maria - Joe's Argentinian wife. Maria is a professional librarian working at a school.

Victoria - Joe and Maria's older daughter.

Teresa - Joe and Maria's younger daughter.

Bill - American living in Argentine for many years and a long-time friend of Joe

Rosario - Bill's Argentinian wife and Maria's best friend since girlhood.

Bill Jr., (Billy) - Bill and Rosario's son.

Dennis - Bill's old college roommate who lives in Miami.

Barbara - Dennis' wife.

Doctor Silva - Joe's long-time family doctor.

Mr. Morgan (South Africa), Mr. Bailey (an Englishman living in Singapore), Mr. Bentley (United States), and Mr. Charles (France) - Proton Therapy patients Joe meets while at the National Cancer Center in Seoul, Korea.

Garza family - friends of Maria and Rosario and acquaintances of Joe, whose son has cancer (Ewing's Sarcoma).

Proton Beam Therapy
for Prostate Cancer

Joe's Presentation to the Rotary Club
Buenos Aires, Argentina

My Story

- Six months ago "prostate" and "prostate cancer" were foreign terms. Then received indication of a problem.
- Five months ago got confirmed diagnosis of prostate cancer; process of learning and deciding.
- Four months ago left for treatment in Korea.
- Returned two months ago.
- Will never be "cured," however disease is now in remission.
- Will have to monitor my condition for the rest of my life.

Prostate Cancer Among Men

- "Old man's disease" saying is not completely true, percentage who have it does increase with age.
- Overall, in the male population, one in six will get prostate cancer.
- Over 200,000 new cases in the US each year (similar to number of new cases for breast cancer).
- Death rate about 15% (breast cancer rate is 19%).

Prostate Cancer

- Higher percentage of older men get it.
- Generally slower developing, so older men more likely to die from another cause.
- Slower developing in about two-thirds of cases.
- Younger men and cases that develop more rapidly require more aggressive response.

What Causes Prostate Cancer?

- No clear indications, as for smoking as cause of lung, mouth, and throat cancers.
- Genetics: If father or brother has it, you are more likely to have it.
- Exploring lifestyle issues, such as diet, but no conclusion yet.

Symptoms

- Urinary dysfunction (frequent need to urinate; painful urination; difficulty maintaining stream or emptying bladder).
- Change in ability to achieve erection.
- Symptoms are similar to those for other conditions, so aren't conclusive indication of cancer.

Methods of Diagnosis

- Most common forms of screening:
  - PSA testing (blood test). Looking for high PSA number or number that is increasing.
  - DRE (Digital Rectal Exam). Looking for prostate "roughness."
- If disease is suspected, following may be done:
  - Biopsy.
  - Bone density scans.
  - MRI.
  - CT scan.

Available Treatments

- "Watchful waiting:" more common if patient is older or suffers other conditions.
- Surgery: remove prostate and other tissue.
- Radiation: ionizes cancer cells (can't reproduce).
  - External (X-ray) radiation ("photon").
  - Internal radiation "brachytherapy," radioactive needles inserted in tumor.
- Chemotherapy.
- Hormone therapy: used to slow growth of tumor.
- Biological therapy.

Side Effects

- Surgery:
  - Damage to sensitive tissues in vicinity of prostate gland.
  - Nearby tissue governs urinary and sexual functions.
- Radiation:
  - Damage to sensitive tissues in vicinity of prostate gland.
  - Radiation must pass through healthy tissue on way to and beyond tumor.
  - Can cause secondary cancers.

Proton Beam Therapy (PBT)

- Beam of charged particles stripped from hydrogen atoms.
- Proton delivers energy to tumor, ionizing cancer cells similar to photon (X-ray) radiation.
- Unique characteristic "Bragg Peak" does not deliver energy until it reaches tumor, where it delivers almost all of its energy.
- Does not affect healthy tissue before or beyond tumor.
- Allows higher doses and minimizes effect on otherwise healthy tissue.

History of Treatment

- Surgery to remove diseases prostate first performed in Tucson in 1893.
- Radiation ionization of cancer cells discovered son after discovery of radiation.
- Proton beam as treatment method theorized after World War II.
- Experiments with proton; practical use required sufficient development of computers.
- Proton in clinical use since 1990.

Proton Beam Therapy Facilities

- Loma Linda University Medical Center (1990).
- Used equipment taken from experimental proton facility.
- Now eleven locations worldwide; nine in the United States.
- Several facilities under construction or under development.

Criteria for Selecting Treatment Facility

- Accessibility: how close/convenient is facility.
- Delay: how soon would treatment be available.
- Qualifications of personnel.
- Advancements in treatment: does the facility keep up with these?
- Cost.
- Intangibles.

Treatment in Korea

- National Cancer Center (NCC)
- About 40% or 50% of cost in US facilities.
- Fully qualified staff – Director is US trained.
- Cost includes apartment and transportation between apartment and NCC for treatment.
- Concierge to help with non-medical arrangements.
- Takes about 8 weeks.

Korea as an Exciting Destination

- Rapidly developing economy and rapidly advancing country.
- Many cultural traditions preserved and available to view.
- Easy to get around.
- Many people speak English.

Summary

- Men should have PSA tested routinely.
- If indications of problem, discuss results with doctor.
- Be aware of health conditions and make wise, informed choices.
- If diagnosed with prostate cancer, investigate if qualify for proton beam therapy.
- If qualify, consider treatment at NCC in Seoul, Korea.

ABOUT THE AUTHORS

York L. Phillips was born in Colorado and has lived in many places in the United States and overseas. He attended the University of Illinois and Virginia Tech. Phillips retired in 2011 from a career as an urban planner, writing ordinances, zoning reports, and similar technical documents for over forty years. Having an interest in writing, Phillips decided to work with Curtis Poling on a book about prostate cancer and proton beam therapy. Other writing projects on the shelf include a play, a novel, and a non-fiction book about the development of a new proton beam center. Phillips is married to Vicki Phillips and resides in coastal Georgia, USA.

Curtis Poling was born in Ohio and has lived in many places in the United States pursuing a career in the building products and home improvement products industries. In 2007, at age 53, Poling was diagnosed with prostate cancer. A thorough person by nature, Poling investigated his options through research on the Internet and discussions with a variety of medical professionals, with particular attention to the adverse effects of the various treatments. Poling discovered proton beam therapy and pursued this option at Loma Linda University Medical Center in California. After overcoming his cancer, Poling began blogging to make others aware of the availability and benefits of proton beam therapy. Poling now serves in the US with KMI International, helping patients from around the world obtain treatment at the National Cancer Center in Seoul, Korea. Poling is married to Tracy Poling and resides in coastal Georgia, USA.

www.ingramcontent.com/pod-product-compliance
Lightning Source LLC
Chambersburg PA
CBHW072249270326
41930CB00010B/2316

* 9 7 8 0 6 1 5 6 4 5 3 6 0 *